Sexually transmitted infections

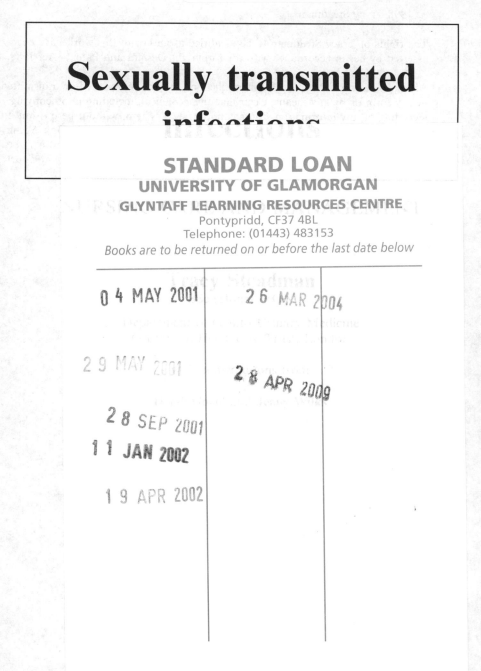

Stanley Thornes (Publishers) Ltd

First published in 1998 by:
Stanley Thornes (Publishers) Ltd
Ellenborough House
Wellington Street
CHELTENHAM
GL50 1YW
United Kingdom

98 99 00 01 02 / 10 9 8 7 6 5 4 3 2 1

A catalogue record for this book is available from the British Library

ISBN 0-7487-3337-X

Typeset by Acorn Bookwork, Salisbury, Wiltshire
Printed in Great Britain by T J International, Padstow, Cornwall

Contents

Acknowledgements

The realization of this book is the end of a long journey with many pitfalls, all at last overcome. Its completion would not have been possible without the determined encouragement of my editor, Rosemary Morris, who kept faith and to whom I am very grateful. I would also like to thank Dinah Gould for her valuable guidance and direct contribution to the book. To Denis Cobell, I am grateful for the opportunity to have drawn on his experience in the field of genitourinary medicine; I value his continued friendship. There are many other people to thank who have helped along the way, particularly Dr Judy Russell, who checked the manuscript for medical accuracy. I would like to thank my family for their unfailing support in everything I do, and lastly, Simon for his love and encouragement without which this project would never have reached completion. I would like to dedicate this book to Ruby Olive Foster, who is no longer with me in body but always in spirit.

The author and publishers would also like to acknowledge the Public Health Laboratory Service for permission to reproduce the graph on page 31. Every effort has been made to contact copyright holders and we apologise if any have been overlooked.

Introduction

The nursing care and management of people with sexually transmitted infections involves specialist skills which appear initially to have little in common with other fields of nursing. Deeper analysis of this speciality, with its particular emphasis on confidentiality, reveals that nursing both adapts and develops its fundamental principles and skills in this setting. Communication skills in particular are applied to gain information, provide education and, in most cases, facilitate self-care. This specialist expertise and its associated clinical skills provide the foundation of a holistic approach to caring for the physical and psychological well-being of patients with sexually transmitted infections.

Although nursing in general has moved away from the traditional role of handmaiden to one of providing individualized care, with an emphasis on communication, some claim this process has gone too far (Webb, 1992). It is acknowledged that psychological care is important, but not at the expense of the traditional skills concerned with physical care and comfort. Salvage (1990) introduced the concept of 'new nursing', defined as the use of models focusing on psychological, social and physical needs. This primary nursing allows nurse and patient to plan care together, thus improving communication, a useful notion in the field of genitourinary (GU) medicine.

Genitourinary medicine (GUM) is a specialized discipline, where nurses have often first gained experience in other specialities. Gynaecology and urology often supply GUM with nurses who have recognized the links between these disciplines and wish to learn more about GUM. Nurses may be attracted to the speciality by chance, having completed a placement, perhaps only a day, in a GUM clinic during training or induction into a related speciality. Even this brief experience of GUM may have demonstrated the unique role of the nurse and the combination of well-developed communication, health education and teamwork skills necessary to achieve competency in this area.

A MODEL FOR GU NURSING

It is rare that a model of nursing is used in GUM, because of the highly specialized nature of the role. To be effective a model should place equal emphasis on psychological, social and physical factors. Some models emphasizing psychological care have been criticized and thought appropriate only for psychiatric nursing. In GUM it could be argued that the psychological and emotional care of individuals is a priority, often surpassing the need for physical care. Orem's model would appear to be the most appropriate, based on the principle that individuals sustain their own health through their own ability to do so. This ability depends upon many factors including maturity, knowledge, life experiences, thought patterns and their physical and mental state. The degree of intervention by the nurse will depend upon the individual's ability to perform self-care, nursing being provided in a complementary relationship to this (Fraser, 1996). Orem's method includes teaching in order to promote self-care, hence the nurse's role in GUM as educator. Unfortunately the adoption of such a complex model is hampered by the fact that many patients attend a GUM clinic only once or twice and for a very short length of time. Perhaps this is an opportunity for GU nurses to devise a helpful and practical model particularly suited for their unique discipline.

The named-nurse concept, as outlined in *The Patient's Charter* (Department of Health, 1992), has been introduced into GUM, with some effect, in an attempt to improve communication as part of the psychological care of the patient. Continuity of care can be achieved when the same nurse assesses, examines, treats and evaluates the patient. This may improve compliance with treatment and encourage attendance at follow-up visits. The named-nurse initiative can be of particular use in the treatment of genital warts, for example.

COMMUNICATION

In genitourinary medicine the emphasis on communication is greater than in many other disciplines of nursing. This is mainly due to the sensitive and confidential nature of the speciality. The establishment of good communication, enabling trusting relationships with patients to be developed, is fundamental to effective care and management (Dickson, Hargie and Morrow, 1997). There have been numerous definitions of communication but for the purposes of this text the definition of Hewes and Planalp (1987) is appropriate. They highlight two main themes. Firstly, intersubjectivity, i.e. striving to understand others and being understood in turn. Secondly, impact, i.e. the extent to which a message can change feelings, thoughts and behaviours. These two themes must be borne in mind in order to communicate effectively with patients.

The nurse in GUM needs to be skilled in eliciting relevant information that will assist in diagnosis, treatment and support of the individual. Tactful probing, respecting boundaries, is a prerequisite skill, and trust is essential for information to be disclosed. The invasion of privacy is a sensitive issue and the extent of self-disclosure depends on the level of reassurance felt by the individual. Any information imparted should be kept in the strictest confidence. A breach of this may result in people defaulting for important follow-up visits. These skills are largely achieved through experience, many GU nurses becoming almost unshockable and gaining a high degree of clinical objectivity. A knowledge of sexuality in all its forms is important and nurses need to be provided with training in order to develop professionally. Discussion and acceptance of cultural and subcultural norms will enable the nurse to communicate on most levels. This is a great advantage in the normalization of disclosed behaviour. Nurses do need to be aware of the danger of complacency and cynicism. Nurses in this field also need support and supervision as they may face many challenging situations. However non-judgemental they believe themselves to be, some disclosures may involve sexual practices that they may find unacceptable, e.g. paedophilia. In addition, in the case of HIV infection, issues of death and dying can be difficult for nurses. With assistance, each nurse will develop coping strategies to deal with these diverse and challenging situations. The author has observed that one such strategy often adopted in GUM is that of humour, which is well recognized as helping to reduce tension.

SCOPE OF PRACTICE AND HEALTH EDUCATION

One of the main features of nursing in GUM is the extended role elements essential to achieve competency in this area. *The Scope of Professional Practice* (United Kingdom Central Council, 1992) supports nurses using initiative and improving their practice on the basis of sound skills and knowledge. The autonomous nature of much of the work attracts many nurses to the discipline because here they can achieve competencies unavailable to them in other areas. These include clinical techniques including microscopy, venepuncture, cervical smear-taking and colposcopy. These skills are gained through training and experience and are used to assist clinical diagnosis.

In addition to the acquisition of clinical skills necessary for competency in this field, the role includes an important function of education and health promotion. Although individuals ultimately have responsibility for their own health and behaviour, the nurse is instrumental in educating individuals to assist them as far as possible to make informed choices. This depends again upon good communication skills, enabling people to understand health messages and to believe they can act upon them. The current level of knowledge must be assessed and then built upon to increase knowledge and understanding. There are many other factors to take into consideration, most importantly societal and individual values, and rules that promote behaviour conducive to health (Webb, 1994). In addition it is important to recognize that the nurse may lack information about the person and their situation, which may present obstacles to effective interaction.

The nurse will give advice and information about safer sexual practices and also broader issues of sexual health, e.g. contraceptive advice, many nurses in GUM being skilled in family planning issues. In many GUM clinics the nurses are expected to advise on self-administered medication and to encourage compliance and follow-up. It is also important for nurses to recognize the limits of their expertise and advise referral to other professionals if appropriate. In a growing number of areas nurses are taking over elements of assessment, diagnosis and the prescription of medication; a role that appears to be an obvious progression for nurses in GUM. An experienced nurse may have many of the qualities of the clinical nurse specialist. The role of the experienced GUM nurse can be likened to the definition of a clinical nurse specialist as a practitioner who shows an advanced level of skill and knowledge while acting as a role model for less experienced nurses, setting standards, giving expert advice to colleagues and teaching (Markham, 1988).

With the increased responsibility and wider scope of practice of the nurse in areas like GUM comes the question of accountability. It is recognized that nurses, even if following orders from medical personnel, are accountable for their own actions (United Kingdom Central Council, 1984). It is the nurse's responsibility that no omission or action on their part is detrimental to the safety or condition of the patient. The nurse in GUM should be encouraged to accept this responsibility, working in close collaboration with other health care professionals (United Kingdom Central Council, 1992).

THE MULTIDISCIPLINARY TEAM

The relationship between doctor and nurse in GUM has evolved into one that in many cases is totally interdependent. This model has gone a long way to eliminate the concept of the subservient nurse and recognize that each health care professional provides essential elements of care. In GUM the concept of teamwork is of utmost importance. The relationship of nurse, doctor, health adviser, clerical staff and other personnel must be integrated and symbiotic in order for the service to function effectively. The battle between the medical and nursing disciplines is largely resolved here, with the recognition of the nurse's role in diagnosis and treatment. Both nurse and doctor have something unique to offer and should be totally interdependent (Faulkner, 1996). Although each member of the team has a distinct role, referral to other team members may have local variations according to the skill mix. The nurse often has a key role in the referral to other personnel.

NURSING RESEARCH

One important way in which nurses may assert authority in a discipline is through undertaking nursing research in that area. In GUM as in most areas there is a lack of nursing research. This is unfortunate in an area where the individuality and experience of the clientele lends itself to investigation and thus the improvement of services and a deeper understanding of the needs of different cultural and social groups. It is known through medical research that the incidence of certain sexually transmitted infections varies with many factors including lifestyle and cultural differences. According to their geography, GUM clinics encounter different problems and needs and the author is convinced that this presents an ideal opportunity for nurses to increase their participation in research to achieve the ultimate goal of continuing improvement of patient care.

I hope that this book will assist nurses in the exciting speciality of GUM to broaden their knowledge of sexually transmitted infections and of the nurse's role in the care of GUM patients. Most specialist nurses in this field derive much satisfaction from the treatability of sexually transmitted infections and the important element of education about sexual health. This book provides the theoretical background for achieving this and hopefully will inspire nurses with confidence to undertake further research into this growing and essential field of nursing.

REFERENCES

Department of Health (1992) *The Patient's Charter: Raising the Standard*, HMSO, London.
Dickson, D., Hargie, O. and Morrow, N. (1997) *Communication Skills Training for Health Professionals*, 2nd edn, Chapman & Hall, London.
Faulkner, A. (1996) *Nursing: The Reflective Approach to Adult Nursing Practice*, 2nd edn, Chapman & Hall, London.
Fraser, M. (1996) *Conceptual Nursing in Practice: A Research-Based Approach*, 2nd edn, Chapman & Hall, London.

Hewes, D. and Planalp, S. (1987) The individual's place in communication science, in *Handbook of Communication Science* (eds C. Berger and S. Chaffee), Sage, London.

Markham, G. (1988) Special cases. *Nursing Times,* **8**(26), 29–30.

Salvage, J. (1990) The theory and practice of the 'new nursing'. *Nursing Times,* **84**(4), 42–5.

United Kingdom Central Council (1984) *Code of Professional Conduct for the Nurse, Midwife and Health Visitor,* UKCC, London.

United Kingdom Central Council (1992) *The Scope of Professional Practice,* UKCC, London.

Webb, C. (1992) What is nursing? *British Journal of Nursing,* **1**(11), 567–8.

Webb, P. (1994) *Health Promotion and Patient Education: A Professional's Guide,* Chapman & Hall, London.

FURTHER READING

Buckeldee, J. (1993) *Nursing Research and Issues,* Chapman & Hall, London.

Ewles, L. and Simnett, I. (1992) *Promoting Health: A Practical Guide,* 2nd edn, Scutari Press, London.

Hardey, M. and Mulhall, A. (1994) *Nursing Research: Theory and Practice,* Chapman & Hall, London.

Kagan, C. (1994) *Professional Interpersonal Skills for Nurses,* 2nd edn, Chapman & Hall, London.

The history of sexually transmitted infections

1

BACKGROUND

Over the past century there has been a decline in the incidence of most infectious diseases in developed countries. Smallpox is extinct. Cholera, diphtheria and poliomyelitis are rare. The incidence of tuberculosis has declined in general, although as a disease of immigrants from developing countries and as an opportunistic infection in immunocompromised patients with HIV and AIDS, it has shown signs of resurgence. Syphilis is no longer common, and responds well to treatment, though gonorrhoea still poses a problem. The incidence of many other sexually transmitted infections, particularly viral infections, continues to increase (see Chapter 3).

The origins of infectious diseases are often not clear due to the former lack of techniques for diagnosis. Historically many diagnoses were made by observation of clinical signs and symptoms.

Syphilis appears to have been unknown in Europe until just before the end of the fifteenth century. It is popularly thought to have been brought to Europe by Columbus' sailors on their return from voyages of discovery to the New World, although there is still argument about evidence gleaned from bones recovered from archaeological sites in the Old World, and from descriptions based on biblical and classical texts, indicating the possible presence of syphilis before the fifteenth century. Infections similar to syphilis are still in evidence today and there is a strong possibility that syphilis is a mutation of bejel, pinta or yaws. Whatever the truth about the origins of syphilis, there is plenty of evidence to suggest that an epidemic of syphilis occurred in Europe in the early years of the sixteenth century. This was the Renaissance period and one of the great scholars of that time, Erasmus (1466–1536), gave a vivid description of syphilis and its effects:

> If I were asked which is the most destructive of all diseases I should unhesitatingly reply that it is that which has been raging with impunity. It combines in itself all the terrible features of other contagions — pain, infection, danger of death, and disagreeable and repugnant treatment which does not produce a complete cure. (quoted in Oriel, 1994)

Fracastoro of Verona (1478–1553), a physician to the Council of Trent, gave an early description of the genital sores associated with syphilis in its early stages and also gave a vivid outline of the effects of the lesions syphilis produced:

> They always broke down in a few days, and constantly discharged an incredible quantity of stinking matter ... those attacked on the upper parts of the body suffered from malignant affectations which ate away sometimes the palate ... the fauces ... the larynx: some lost their lips, some their nose, others all their genital organs. Many had gummatous tumours on the limbs which were often the size of an egg. (Fracastoro, 1546)

The recognition of various manifestations of syphilis in the body evolved slowly between the sixteenth and eighteenth centuries. Ambroise Pare, an illustrious French surgeon, refers to early treatments for syphilis such as inunctions of mercury or guaiacum and sulphur baths (Cobell, 1965). William Clowes (1504–1604) was a surgeon at St Batholomew's hospital, who wrote about the cure of syphilis by the use of unctions and, as was common among writers of the time, criticised in unbridled terms, those suffering from syphilis — an early indication of the stigma attached to sexually transmitted infections.

A number of prominent figures in medical history also appear in the history of sexually transmitted infections. The first adequate account of the primary chancre of syphilis was given by John Hunter (1728–1793). In 1767, after he experimentally inoculated himself with gonorrhoea that was contaminated with syphilitic spirochetes, he developed a chancre and concluded that gonorrhoea and syphilis were the same disease. His theory was that syphilis was caused by an organism landing on a cutaneous membrane, and gonorrhoea was caused by an organism landing on a mucous membrane. This view lasted until Benjamin Bell (1749–1805) published his *Treatise on Gonorrhoea Virulenta and Lues Venerea* in 1793, which concluded the separation of gonorrhoea and syphilis on the grounds that their signs and symptoms were dissimilar, that gonorrhoea does not progress to syphilis, and that treatment for one disease was ineffective in curing the other.

The advent of the modern approach to syphilis diagnosis came with Philippe Ricord (1800–1899). He outlined the stages of syphilis and also noted the transmission by homosexual contact. Jonathon Hutchinson (1828–1913), an eminent figure in nineteenth-century England, engaged in further research on syphilis. He is chiefly remembered for his description of congenital syphilis, which included interstitial keratitis, labyrinthine deafness and notched peg-shaped permanent incisors. He warned those in his profession about differential diagnosis in a famous paper on syphilis as the great imitator.

DIAGNOSIS OF SEXUALLY TRANSMITTED INFECTIONS

The precise diagnosis of diseases such as gonorrhoea and syphilis had to wait for the construction of microscopes of sufficient magnification and resolution, and later serological tests. Alexandre Donne (1801–1878) published a paper in 1836 about various genitourinary discharges in both sexes, having seen organisms similar to vibrios in material isolated from a chancre.

Fritz Schaudinn (1871–1906) and Eric Hoffman (1868–1959) discovered *Treponema pallidum* in Berlin in 1905. They saw the pale spiral organisms rotating and flexing on their axis from material obtained from a vulval papule of a young woman. This was also identified by the same workers in stained preparations from other patients with early syphilis.

In 1906 Wasserman (1866–1925) established a serological test for syphilis. This showed that there were complement-fixing antibodies which could be identified in sera in the laboratory.

In earlier times the discharge of gonorrhoea had been confused with seminal fluid and indeed the term 'gonorrhoea' derives from the Greek for 'flowing from seed'. The confusion continued until Albert Neisser (1855–1916) clarified the situation by applying Koch's postulates. Koch (1843–1910) had established stains for bacteria and developed a medium for growing them. He had also laid down what later became known as 'Koch's postulates'. These were:

1. Bacteria should be present in every case of disease.
2. It should be possible to grow the bacteria on a medium.
3. The culture should be able to reproduce the disease when re-inoculated.

Treponema pallidum is one of the few bacteria that do not fulfil Koch's postulates as it cannot grow on media.

Initially Neisser used Koch's staining techniques, employing methyl blue. He noticed that the bacteria isolated from purulent urethral and vaginal discharges always appeared in pairs. Neisser, whose name was to become associated with this bacterium, *Neisseria gonorrhoeae*, later used the method of Danish microbiologist Gram, and observed that gonococci were the only organisms to appear in gonococcal pus and did not appear in any other disease.

TREATMENTS FOR SEXUALLY TRANSMITTED INFECTIONS

Before the development of modern treatment, there was a variety of remedies for syphilis and other sexually transmitted disease. Urethral and vaginal discharges were often treated by irrigations and douches — a solution of weak potassium permanganate often being used, and still used today for some conditions.

Syphilis was treated by applications of compounds or by systemic medicines: compounds containing mercury or iodides, but also naturalistic remedies such as guaiacum — a herbal treatment from the West Indies. Fever therapy was not uncommon; this consisted of attempting to raise the patient's temperature to diminish the effect the bacteria may have on the body.

Paul Ehrlich (1854–1955) performed many experiments with compounds of arsenic. In 1909 his experimentation led to the use of arsephenamine, known as 606, which was found to have some effect. Later bismuth was used.

Alexander Fleming (1881–1955) discovered penicillin in 1928, but it was not until the 1940s that it was developed into an antimicrobial treatment. It has since remained the drug of choice in the treatment of syphilis and gonorrhoea.

ATTITUDES TO SEXUAL HEALTH

Some of the historical references quoted in this chapter demonstrate that attitudes to sexually transmitted infections did not begin to change until relatively recently. Attitudes were particularly severe under the Victorian patriarchs, demonstrated when some parts of Shakespeare's works were excluded as they were considered indelicate or profane. Venereal diseases, as they were known then, were categorized under a series of Contagious Diseases Acts in the 1860s which compelled prostitutes in dock and army garrison towns to register and be medically examined (Ferris, 1993). The attitude that sexually transmitted infections were a great evil scourge or plague was rife. As with every plague the population felt the need to identify a group who were responsible. Inevitably those members of society who were viewed as outsiders, whether because of difference in ethnicity, religion or sexual orientation, were blamed for the spread of disease (Sontag, 1989).

In 1916 a Commission on Venereal Diseases was set up in response to the enormous increase in cases of gonorrhoea and syphilis in the First World War; this was the forerunner to setting up today's modern, free, confidential service for diagnosis and treatment of sexually transmitted infections. Among its members were clergy and moralists, who saw it as their duty to stamp out diseases by imposing strict rules governing sexual behaviour. Condoms became more readily available although they were not widely spoken of. Once penicillin became available for the treatment of syphilis and gonorrhoea, attitudes to sexual health slowly began to change.

After the Second World War, and a similar increase in sexually transmitted infections, the network of clinics in the United Kingdom was taken over by the National Health Service in 1948. In essence these services remain today, although they have expanded greatly due to the changing patterns of sexually transmitted infections (see Chapter 2).

Although the network of GU services is now well established in the United Kingdom and has done much to reduce the stigma of sexually transmitted infections, unfortunately the 'plague' mentality and discrimination still exist in many parts of society today. With the advent of HIV, many of the historical attitudes towards those with sexually transmitted infections were rekindled and blame was directed at those seen to be marginal members of society. The theory that HIV originated in Africa was convenient for those who apportioned blame according to racial differences. Similarly the rapid increase in incidence of HIV amongst homosexual men added fuel to those of the opinion that 'deviant' sexual behaviour had to be followed by some kind of divine retribution (Schafer, 1991). Media coverage of the HIV epidemic, has in many cases only added to the marginalization of certain groups in society by using them as scapegoats. Negative attitudes to sexually transmitted infections have social consequences in terms of the reduction and prevention of these infections as well as impacting on the psychological sequelae of affected individuals.

NURSES' ATTITUDES TO SEXUALLY TRANSMITTED INFECTIONS

With the advent of HIV, health care professionals had real concerns for their safety when caring for people with this new disease. In the early days of HIV many nurses were reluctant to treat people with this infection and all health care professionals sometimes used inappropriate precautions and isolation techniques. These attitudes were inevitable because so little was known about this potentially fatal infection. The belief was that attitudes would improve as nurses were educated and became more knowledgeable about the infection. To a certain extent this was true: regular education and clear guidelines on recommended infection control precautions appeared to reduce fear among nurses working with people with HIV (Malik-Nitto and Plantemoli, 1986).

Unfortunately, inappropriate behaviours and opinions persisted, especially in those nurses not directly working with people with HIV, and against people with HIV in general (Rose and Platzer, 1993). Much of the prejudice was not due to HIV itself but often to the mode of transmission. Negative attitudes were associated with homophobia, intravenous drug use and the fear of death and dying; actual knowledge about HIV was sometimes minimal (Robbins, Cooper and Bender, 1992).

Negative attitudes of nurses towards HIV and other sexually transmitted infections have consequences for nursing care and clients' use of services. It could be argued that such attitudes could have a significant influence on public perceptions, affecting both service use and the effectiveness of prevention programmes — often said to be a key nursing role. An example of this may be that many gay people access those central London GUM clinics where they perceive they will meet with greater tolerance — which is creating a consumer-led service. This may lead to further marginalization of some sections of society; GUM clinics should instead be a catalyst for education and change in nurses' attitudes. Unfortunately, if those who are at the front line of care display negative attitudes and opinions, the rest of society will have a long way to go to achieve a supportive, non-judgemental environment for those affected by sexually transmitted infections.

Nurses, because of their relatively close relationships with those they care for, are in a unique position to act as advocates against prejudice and discrimination and to reduce the stigma associated with sexually transmitted infections. In addition they are ideally placed to advise on ways in which accessibility to services can be improved and to promote a more user-friendly approach (Cranfield, 1996). Genitourinary medicine services need to be innovative and diverse in order to meet the needs of marginalized groups and of other individuals who find it difficult to access services. Nurses have an important part to play in the formulation of strategies to reduce inequalities of access to services.

REFERENCES

Cobell, D. (1965) The origin and history of syphilis. *Nursing Mirror*, **120**, 192–9.

Cranfield, S. (1996) Reducing inequality of access and care provision for people affected by HIV/AIDS, in *AIDS and HIV: The Nursing Response* (eds J. Faugier and I. Hicken), Chapman & Hall, London.

Ferris, P. (1993) *Sex and the British: A Twentieth Century History*, Michael Joseph, London.

Fracastoro, G. (1546) De Morbis Contagiosis, Venice. Quoted in Lanceraux, E. (1868) *A Treatise on Syphilis*, Vol. 1 (trans. G. Whitley), New Sydenham Society, London, 25–6.

Malik-Nitto, S. and Plantemoli, L. (1986) A strategic plan for the management of patients with AIDS. *Nursing Management*, **17**(6), 46–8.

Oriel, J.D. (1994) *The Scars of Venus*, Springer-Verlag, London.

Robbins, I., Cooper, A. and Bender, M.P. (1992) The relationship between knowledge, attitudes and degree of contact with HIV and AIDS. *Journal of Advanced Nursing*, **17**, 198–203.

Rose, P. and Platzer, H. (1993) Confronting Prejudice. *Nursing Times* **49**(31), 52–4.

Schafer, A. (1991) AIDS: the social dimension, in *Perspectives on AIDS: Ethical and Social Issues* (eds C. Overall and W.P. Zion), Oxford University Press, Toronto.

Sontag, S. (1989) *AIDS And Its Metaphors*, Allen Lane / Penguin Press, London.

FURTHER READING

Faugier, J. and Hicken, I. (eds) (1996) *AIDS and HIV: The Nursing Response*, Chapman & Hall, London.

Overall, C. and Zion, W.P. (eds) (1991) *Perspectives on AIDS: Ethical and Social Issues*, Oxford University Press, Toronto.

2 | Structure and scope of genitourinary medicine services

OBJECTIVES

1. To understand the importance of confidentiality.
2. To recognize the changing structure of genitourinary medicine services in response to the increased prevalence of viral infections and to government policy and initiatives on sexual health.
3. To recognize the variations in GU services and recommendations for good practice.
4. To understand the roles of the nurse and all other disciplines of staff represented in GUM.

INTRODUCTION

Due to the enormous increase in cases of gonorrhoea and syphilis during the First World War, highlighted by a report of a Royal Commission on Venereal Diseases in 1916, a network of clinics was set up in the United Kingdom. These services were taken over by the National Health Service (NHS) in 1948, to provide confidential, free and accessible diagnosis and treatment of sexually transmitted infections (STIs). Essentially the same system remains today although GU services have been forced to adapt to the changing pattern of sexually transmitted infections, particularly the increasing prevalence of viral infections, and to government policy and initiatives on sexual health and the provision of health care in general. The scope of GUM has expanded to include the management of a wide range of sexual health problems in addition to the traditional management of sexually transmitted infections, although this is not widely recognized. A recent study demonstrated a troubling lack of understanding among non-GUM health care professionals about the organization of

GU services (McClean, Reid and Scoular, 1996). This highlights the need for GU clinics to provide information about the scope of their services and to improve liaison with other service providers in order to help reduce stigma and encourage a collaborative approach to sexual health.

This chapter describes the structure of GU services in the United Kingdom and how this is adapting in response to the changing face of health care as a whole. The impact of the increasing prevalence of viral infections such as HIV is discussed and also the expanding role of GUM, for example, to include the provision of cervical screening and colposcopy services.

The staffing structure in GUM clinics is multidisciplinary. The nurse's role within this is discussed in this chapter, with emphasis on the importance of teamwork in providing a comprehensive and efficient service.

CONFIDENTIALITY

Confidentiality is one of the prime concerns of all staff dealing with individuals attending GUM clinics. Indeed all patients accessing any health care service are entitled to the strictest confidentiality. Staff in GUM clinics must abide by the regulations laid down in 1974 which specifically cover clients' right to confidentiality. They state that all steps should be taken to:

> Secure any information capable of identifying an individual ... with respect to persons examined or treated for any sexually transmitted disease shall not be disclosed except for the purpose of communicating that information to a medical practitioner, or a person employed under the direction of a medical practitioner in connection with the treatment of persons suffering from such disease or the prevention of the spread thereof. (National Health Service, 1974)

For nurses in any area, confidentiality is recognized as a key issue by the United Kingdom Central Council for Nursing, Midwifery and Health Visiting, who state that:

> Each registered nurse, midwife and health visitor is accountable for his or her practice, and, in the exercise of professional accountability shall: Respect confidential information obtained in the course of professional practice and refrain from disclosing such information without the consent of the patient/client, or a person entitled to act on his/her behalf, except where disclosure is required by law or by the order of a court or is necessary in the public interest. (United Kingdom Central Council, 1987)

The General Medical Council have similar guidance for medical staff.

Confidentiality is important to all individuals attending a GUM clinic. However, it is of particular concern for young people, many of whom may be under sixteen. The right of these young people to confidentiality has evoked recent discussion, leading to the publication of a guidance document to clarify some of the contentious issues (British Medical Association, 1994). It is now agreed in the United Kingdom that a young person is entitled to the same confidentiality as any other person and that health professionals can provide advice and treatment to individuals under sixteen without parental consent. In these instances health professionals must be satisfied that the individual understands the situation and can give consent to any advice, treatment and examinations that may be necessary. This is particularly important in GUM clinics, where individuals may have sexually transmitted infections needing urgent treatment with potentially serious consequences if left untreated. If young people fear that their confidentiality will be breached, they may be reluctant to access the service.

In rare cases a breach of confidentiality may be justified, for example, if the health professional believes that the individual is being sexually abused. In such a case the situation should be discussed with the individual and voluntary disclosure encouraged. If the health professional feels that they must disclose information to, say, social services or the police, they must inform the individual and take full responsibility for their actions.

In order to help reduce the stigma attached to GUM clinics, individuals must feel reassured that any information disclosed to staff will remain in the strictest confidence. In GUM in particular, a breach of confidentiality may have serious consequences for the patient, with the possibility of the person responsible facing disciplinary action.

THE IMPACT OF THE CHANGING STRUCTURE OF THE NATIONAL HEALTH SERVICE ON GU SERVICES

GUM services in the United Kingdom have not only been forced to adapt to the changing patterns of sexually transmitted infections but also to the changing face of health care in general. The structure of the National Health Service has altered immeasurably over the last twenty years, with various government initiatives affecting the way the public access and receive health care services.

Genitourinary medicine clinics provide an open-access self-referral service. This means that people can visit their local clinic or one much further away if they prefer. In 1988 recommendations for the restructuring of the NHS resulted in a White Paper proposing a greater choice of services for patients. This seemed to fit in with the philosophy of GUM.

When the concept of contracting was introduced into the NHS, special arrangements were made with accident and emergency departments to provide care for patients irrespective of their district of residence. It was believed that GU services would operate in a similar way but the situation was by no means clear. Moreover, in order for confidentiality to be maintained it would be difficult to charge the patient's district of residence for a hospital stay as is the case for a patient admitted via accident and emergency. This might happen in the case of HIV patients who may not attend their local GUM clinic.

The following issues were discussed in parliament:

1. The recognition that district health authorities would have to take into account self-referral services for anyone. This in itself does not encourage authorities to provide GU services, as all their residents could use another authority's service.
2. The Monks Report countered this by recommending that GU services be provided in all districts.
3. There was an assurance that no information would be passed to the patient's own health authority.

THE CHANGING STRUCTURE OF GENITOURINARY MEDICINE SERVICES

The comprehensive network of services established from 1948 was effective in controlling the prevalence of infections such as gonorrhoea and syphilis. These services have expanded to deal with all aspects of sexual health. More recently, as the prevalence of bacterial infections has fallen, viral infections such as genital warts and herpes have become increasingly challenging. Management of the viral infections is difficult and time consuming for various reasons:

- Diagnosis can be more difficult.
- Treatment is less satisfactory.
- The implications for the individual and their contacts may be more serious.
- Viral infections often have a longer incubation period, therefore contact tracing can prove difficult.
- In recent years patients have become better informed and may have higher expectations of services.

The epidemiology of both bacterial and viral infections is discussed in Chapter 3.

In the past decade the discovery of HIV has caused the structure of GUM services to change almost beyond recognition. The Department of Health set up an AIDS unit in 1986 which took on responsibility for developing a strategic approach to HIV and AIDS (Department of Health, 1993a). Earmarked funding became available and many GUM clinics have become the centres for HIV testing and counselling and for the management of people with HIV and AIDS. The aim was to limit the further spread of HIV and to provide diagnostic treatment and counselling facilities for those infected or at risk (Department of Health, 1992a). Funding was made available for three main areas:

1. Non-treatment services – HIV prevention.
2. Drug misuse services.
3. Treatment and care costs. This is calculated from the number of live AIDS cases treated in each centre the previous year.

There are several problems with the way this funding is calculated, for example, the difference in requirements between rural and inner-city areas, and the skewed figures caused by improved treatments slowing the progression from HIV to AIDS.

Genitourinary services are in a unique position in the changing climate of the NHS. Rather than competing for contracts and patients, many centres may find themselves overcrowded and unable to cope with the demand. This demand cannot be controlled by contractual constraints and inevitably the inner-city HIV and AIDS treatment centres attract a large proportion of the patients, for the following reasons (Bentley and Adler, 1991):

1. Increased accessibility.
2. Acceptability, due to a number of factors:

   • perceived superior knowledge and skills
   • reputations of professional staff
   • availability of the latest drugs and treatments
   • increased availability of support agencies

3. Assured anonymity.

With the inevitable ending of earmarked funding and the growing importance of commissioning in the National Health Service, GU services need to take note of these developments if they are to play an influential part in recognizing and meeting future sexual health care needs (Evans, Woodward and Patel, 1996). At present the funding allows the provision of a comprehensive sexual health service; however, it is important that this standard of service is maintained and the service does not return to its former status as a 'Cinderella' speciality.

THE FUTURE OF GENITOURINARY MEDICINE SERVICES

In 1992 the government published *The Health of the Nation* (Department of Health, 1992b), which proposed the development of a health strategy for England. This initiative was of particular relevance to GUM in regard to its public health role. As well as outlining several main objectives including the strategic roles of health authorities and the balance between prevention and clinical care, this document proposed key areas to be prioritized for health improvement. One of these key areas was sexual health and HIV/AIDS. Some objectives were laid down:

- To reduce the incidence of HIV and other sexually transmitted infections, specifically gonorrhoea (see Chapter 7).
- To develop monitoring and surveillance of these infections.
- To provide effective services for diagnosis and treatment of these infections.
- To reduce the number of unwanted pregnancies.
- To provide effective family planning services.

One of the main target areas of this document was cervical cancer, the objective being the reduction of incidence of invasive cervical cancer by at least 20% by the year 2000. This has obvious implications for GU services as many women attend for cervical screening and this is one area where the speciality can be seen to contribute to meeting the objectives of this initiative.

According to the document, preventative medicine in general appears to be a clear priority for the government and GUM will play a major part in this co-ordinated, collaborative health strategy.

Nursing's contribution to meeting the targets of *The Health of the Nation* is recognized and the document comprehensively addresses the subjects of HIV/AIDS and sexual health. In a follow-on document (Department of Health, 1993b) clear guidelines were given on ways in which nurses can assist in meeting the government targets. These included:

- improving awareness and knowledge about sexual health, including HIV/AIDS and STIs among local and specific population groups;
- encouraging a safer pattern of sexual behaviour.

This in turn should help to reduce the incidence of HIV, STIs and unwanted pregnancies and maintain high-quality services for the diagnosis and treatment of HIV and other sexually transmitted infections. Nurses in GUM have the expertise and ability to play a major role in meeting government targets for health and in doing so improve the profile of their speciality. Unfortunately the work of nurses in GUM is often poorly understood and hence undervalued. The nursing expertise present in this speciality should be a recognized skill that is used to its full potential.

WORKLOAD IN GUM CLINICS

Due to the increase in the number of cases of HIV and other viral infections the Secretary of State for Social Services initiated a study on the ways in which GUM departments were dealing with this pressure. The final report became known as the Monks Report (Department of Health, 1988).

A working party was set up with the following aims:

1. To examine current and predicted workloads in GUM clinics.
2. To recommend action needed regarding manpower, training, resources and accommodation.

In 1988 the team visited 10% of the clinics in England, at least one in every region, and the following details were examined in each clinic:

- accommodation
- potential for expansion
- staff
- equipment
- support services
- counselling
- flexibility of appointment system
- coordination
- future plans

In this chapter each of these is considered with reference to the Monks Report.

Accommodation

The quality of premises of GUM clinics varies enormously. Traditionally these clinics were very basic, often hidden away in the basement or in temporary accommodation because of the stigma attached to sexually transmitted infections. Unfortunately, this type of accommodation did nothing to improve the image of GUM, and the housing of some clinics today still leaves much to be desired. Poorly designed clinics reduce efficiency and waste staff time.

The Monks Report's recommendations on the housing of GUM clinics are as follows:

1. Clinics should be in the general outpatient department of a hospital.
2. Clinics should be clearly signposted as people may not want to ask directions nor to waste time trying to locate premises.
3. The standard of premises should be not less than that recommended in the Outpatients Department Health Building Note 12 (1988 edition).

4. Areas used for counselling and discussion of confidential matters should be sound-proofed, an important priority in GUM.

Unfortunately it was later observed that in many centres these recommendations were still to be put in place (Allen and Hogg, 1993).

Potential for expansion

Not all GUM clinics are able to expand existing departments. Earmarked funding arrangements have made it possible for some departments to build new accommodation or make alterations to existing premises.

Equipment

The Monks Report observed that provision of equipment in GUM clinics was not a matter of great concern. However, three main areas needed some attention:

1. The need for computerization of clinic records in order to produce data on diagnoses and for audit purposes.
2. Direct telephone lines and prerecorded messages for out of hours information are recommended.
3. Equipment for colposcopy should be considered.

Diagnostic support services

Laboratory support services are essential for the efficient running of GUM clinics. It is recommended that high-quality support is maintained at a level that will meet demand.

Counselling

This is carried out mainly by the health advisers, usually on a one to one basis. Some clinics employ clinical psychologists or psychiatrists on a sessional basis. This is recommended for all GUM clinics.

The Monks Report observed that the quality of counselling services for people with GU problems and those wanting HIV testing was good and recommended that this should continue.

Appointment flexibility

This varies from clinic to clinic and is determined by the type of system used. Walk-in services ensure that there is no waiting time for appointments but can result in overcrowding and long delays. Alternatively, appointment systems ensure that each patient has an allotted amount of time but waiting lists can be problematic. Long waiting lists are unacceptable as this may lead to spread of infection and complications. It is recommended that anyone presenting to a GUM clinic with a suspected sexually transmitted infection should be seen the same day or the next time the clinic is open.

Another consideration is the provision of services outside working hours and it is recommended that some clinic sessions are held after 5 p.m.

Co-ordination

The Monks Report highlighted the need for management and consultants to co-ordinate services in order to prepare for the projected epidemic of HIV. This has occurred to some extent even though the rise in number of new cases of HIV infection is not as high as was initially predicted.

Future plans

When the Monks Report was published there was concern about funding for HIV services and the allocation of this funding to GUM clinics. To a great extent GUM clinics have benefited from this provision and have largely met the recommendations that there should be GU and HIV provision in every district. Additional resources were provided to improve services and staffing levels but GUM clinics must consolidate their position in the event that the earmarked funding is reduced.

STAFFING STRUCTURE AND ROLES IN GUM CLINICS

The staffing structure of clinics appears to be similar throughout the United Kingdom, the basic complement of staff consisting of:

- nursing staff
- medical staff
- health advisers
- receptionists
- secretaries

Other staff may also work closely with the clinics:

- psychologist
- clinical nurse specialist
- social worker
- dietitian
- pharmacist
- palliative care team

THE ROLE OF THE NURSE

The role of the nurse in GUM varies enormously. There appears to be a great diversity in the amount of responsibility nurses have in this speciality. The Monks Report found that the level of responsibility 'does not necessarily reflect the experience of the staff but rather local custom and practice'. In some clinics the specialist skills of nurses appeared underused whereas in others the nurses accepted an inappropriate burden of responsibility. For example, in some clinics new patients were examined by a nurse, some with little medical support. The Monks Report clearly recommends that all new patients be examined by a doctor as is the accepted practice in the United Kingdom. This may change if a nurse practitioner system is fully developed and established. At present it is appropriate for patients attending clinics for follow-up to be assessed and examined by nurses according to agreed local guidelines.

A study by Allen and Hogg (1993) observed the nurse's role in GUM by visiting 20 GUM clinics and interviewing all disciplines of staff represented. Many nurses felt that they had insufficient responsibility and that they would like to widen their role in the clinic. A large proportion would have liked to develop their counselling skills and those who did not participate in microscopy and colposcopy felt that this would be beneficial both for their own professional development and for users of the service.

In some GUM clinics nurse-led clinics run alongside the doctors' clinics. Nurses taking on such a role must be competent according to the guidelines of the United Kingdom Central Council (1992) and accountable for their actions. In addition, nursing documentation must be of a high standard as a means of communication to the multidisciplinary team and as an accurate record of nursing intervention (United Kingdom Central Council, 1993).

Male and female examination

The role of the nurse in GUM clinics is determined to some extent by the sex of the clients they are dealing with. Nurses treating male patients will have a larger role to play in examination, diagnosis and treatment. Those nursing female patients may in some cases be largely acting as a chaperone for the doctor. The main reason for this is anatomy. With women the procedure is more complex, including a bimanual examination. Currently very few nurses are trained to carry out this procedure, so it remains under the remit of the medical staff. This is an area of development for nurses in GUM and recent guidelines laid down by the Royal College of Nursing (1995) will assist nurses in gaining expertise in this procedure.

An important and often undervalued role of the nurse is that of providing comfort for people undergoing intimate examinations. If the experience of examination is made as comfortable as possible, there may be an increased likelihood that the patient will return to the clinic for follow-up visits. This is also important in encouraging attendance, as patient satisfaction with the service will travel by word of mouth and encourage others to attend.

In many clinics nurses will undertake the examination of female patients on follow-up visits. This may include cervical smear testing and chlamydia and gonorrhoea diagnosis.

Microscopy

In many clinics nurses carry out microscopy for both male and female patients (see Chapter 17). Historically this task was carried out by GU technicians who were not trained nurses. In some clinics this was taken over by laboratory technicians or medical staff. It would appear that this is an area where nurses can gain knowledge and expertise and provide continuity of care.

Treatment of genital warts

In most GUM clinics the management and treatment of genital warts is a well established part of the nurse's role. The diagnosis will be made on the first visit to the clinic and then the nurse will take over the management. The patient will be referred back to the doctor at intervals for review of the treatment. This is an area where many nurses have become expert practitioners and are responsible for the assessment and selection of appropriate treatment. A variety of treatments are used by nurses including cryotherapy (see Chapter 11).

Venepuncture

In most GUM clinics it is the nurses who perform venepuncture. This contributes to good continuity of care and enables the nurse to develop the high degree of expertise and skill needed to perform this procedure safely and efficiently (see Chapter 17).

Counselling

Although in the majority of GUM clinics counselling is the remit of health advisers, nurses are also involved to some extent. Much of the nurse's time is spent in reassuring patients who are understandably anxious and in providing psychological care. Some nurses engage in pre-test and post-test counselling for HIV testing and inevitably are involved in the psychological care of individuals affected by HIV and AIDS and other sexually transmitted infections.

In addition, patient education and the explanation of examinations and results is an integral part of providing people with a holistic, quality standard of nursing care. By empowering patients in this way, nurses can assist in increasing the patient's feeling of control over the situation and can promote understanding of and compliance with treatment. The nurse is in an ideal position to take opportunities for patient education on a whole range of issues.

Training is required to enable nurses to develop professionally and achieve competency in the skills necessary to provide a high standard of care to people with sexually transmitted infections. The Monks Report highlighted the need for the review of specialist courses for nurses in GUM as they were found to be often outdated and inaccessible. For further discussion and information on the role of nurses in GUM and on nursing procedures and competencies, see Chapter 17.

THE ROLE OF THE MEDICAL STAFF

In most departments of GUM a consultant will lead the medical team, which will vary in size according to the size and location of the clinic. It may consist of several consultants or just one, and other junior doctors. In many clinics, clinical assistants will work on a sessional basis. These are usually local GPs or GU specialists who prefer to work on a locum circuit.

In recent years the speciality has attracted younger and increasingly dynamic medical interest, which can be mainly attributed to the advent of HIV. This has enabled the speciality to expand its expertise.

The structure of the medical staffing within GUM clinics does much to determine the roles and function of the other members of the team. Unfortunately in the past this often depended on the personality of the consultant. Recently, as nurses have become more autonomous and developed their own areas of expertise, the hierarchy has diminished.

THE ROLE OF THE HEALTH ADVISER

Health advisers have varied backgrounds: many have a nursing qualification; some a social work or health education background. It has been observed that the counselling component of the work is the main attraction to health advising. Other reasons for entering this role are the contact with patients and interest in HIV and AIDS (Allen and Hogg, 1993).

In the study by Allen and Hogg (1993) health advisers stated their main roles as follows.

Education

This relates to education about safe sex and about sexually transmitted infections including HIV and AIDS.

Counselling

This is obviously a key role. It includes counselling on general issues as well as pre-test and post-test counselling for HIV.

Contact tracing and partner notification

Contact tracing in the UK was established over 40 years ago, to identify, diagnose and treat contacts of persons with venereal diseases. It remains a fundamental strategy in the control of STIs today (Shastd, 1992). With the advent of HIV, partner notification and contact-tracing strategies have evoked discussion but they are recognized to be fraught with difficulties (Wright, 1996). For further discussion see Chapter 16.

Training other health professionals

Generally health advisers do not see every person who attends a GUM clinic. Usually selected patients are referred because:

- They have been diagnosed with a sexually transmitted infection, such as gonorrhoea, syphilis, chlamydia, herpes.
- They are considering testing for HIV.
- They need additional support, advice or education.
- They require ongoing counselling because they are HIV positive.

The role of the health adviser is often unclearly defined and differs from clinic to clinic. The training of health advisers has been inconsistent and needs to be rationalized. In addition it is difficult to measure the effectiveness of the work of health advisers, as in most counselling disciplines. Because it cannot be measured quantitatively, members of the profession can often feel undervalued.

Several recommendations emerged from the Monks Report about the role of health advisers:

- Every clinic should have at least one health adviser.

- Certificated courses for health advisers should be established. These are beginning to become evident.
- The professional status of health advisers should be recognized.

THE ROLE OF ADMINISTRATIVE AND CLERICAL STAFF

This group of staff are important in GUM clinics because they are often the first point of contact with the clinic and therefore create the first impression of a speciality that is often feared.

Documentation and note keeping are particularly important in GUM, given the nature of the information. It is therefore important that filing systems are maintained efficiently. In addition the clerical staff often assist in the monitoring of attendances and diagnoses to provide epidemiological data.

The importance of this discipline of staff is often underestimated. The job can be challenging, many receptionists often having to deal with aggressive or anxious patients.

The emphasis has moved towards teamwork and the realisation that for a department to function efficiently the different expertise of each discipline of staff must be acknowledged. Each discipline has unique skills and a part to play in service provision. The image of GUM has improved but negative attitudes and stigma still prevail. It is this multidisciplinary approach and the consequent provision of high-quality care which will further raise the profile of GU services and the professionals working in this field. The ultimate aims are to eliminate the stigma of sexually transmitted infections and to demand recognition for the unique expertise required to provide such a service.

REFERENCES

Allen, I. and Hogg, D. (1993) *Work Roles and Responsibilities in Genitourinary Medicine Clinics*, Policy Studies Institute, London.

Bentley, C. and Adler, M.W. (1991) Genitourinary medicine, AIDS and the NHS Act: will contracting arrangements lead to contracted services? *Genitourinary Medicine*, **67**(1), 10–14.

British Medical Association (1994) *Confidentiality and People Under 16*, BMA, London.

Department of Health (1988) *Report of the Working Group to Examine Workloads in Genitourinary Medicine Clinics* (The Monks Report), DOH, London.

Department of Health (1992a) *AIDS Briefing Note*. DOH, London.

Department of Health (1992b) *The Health of the Nation: A Strategy for Health for England*, HMSO, London.

Department of Health (1993a) *Government Strategy on HIV and AIDS*. DOH, London.

Department of Health (1993b) *Targeting Practice: The Contribution of Nurses, Midwives and Health Visitors*, DOH, London.

Evans, D., Woodward, N. and Patel, R. (1996) Commissioning genitourinary medicine services: the policy research agenda. *International Journal of STD & AIDS*, **7**(2), 87–90

McClean, H.L., Reid, R. and Scoular, A. (1996) 'Healthy Alliances?' – other sexual health services and their views of genitourinary medicine. *Genitourinary Medicine*, **71**(6), 396–9

National Health Service (1974) *The National Health Service (Venereal Diseases) Regulations*, HMSO, London.

Royal College of Nursing (1995) *Bimanual Pelvic Examination: Guidance for Nurses*, RCN, London.

The Society of Health Advisers in Sexually Transmitted Diseases (Shastd) (1992) Partner Notification Guidelines. MSF.

United Kingdom Central Council (1987) *Confidentiality. An elaboration of Clause 9 of the Second Edition of the UKCC's Code of Professional Conduct for the Nurse, Midwife and Health Visitor*, UKCC, London.

United Kingdom Central Council (1992) *The Scope of Professional Practice*, UKCC, London.

United Kingdom Central Council (1993) *Standards for Records and Record Keeping*, UKCC, London.

Wright, S. (1996) AIDS: ethical dilemmas and the nursing response, in *AIDS and HIV: The Nursing Response* (eds J. Faugier and I. Hicken), Chapman & Hall, London, pp. 46–70.

FURTHER READING

Faugier, J. and Hicken, I. (eds) (1996) *AIDS and HIV: The Nursing Response*, Chapman & Hall, London.

Levitt, R., Wall. A. and Appleby, J. (1995) *The Reorganized National Health Service*, 5th edn, Chapman & Hall, London.

Epidemiology of sexually transmitted infections

3

OBJECTIVES

1. To understand the importance of the epidemiology of sexually transmitted infections and the implications for prevention strategies.
2. To describe the development of epidemiological research and surveillance in GUM.
3. To understand the two main strategies for prevention and control of
sexually transmitted infections: contact tracing and health education.
4. To become familiar with the basic epidemiology of each sexually transmitted infection.
5. To describe the reporting systems used by GU clinics in the United
Kingdom.

INTRODUCTION

According to Meers, Sedgwick and Worsley (1995), 'epidemiology is the
science of the study and control of epidemic diseases'. This definition can
be expanded to include the study of the rate of spread of diseases, known
as the 'incidence'. In addition the 'prevalence' is the number of people
suffering from a condition at any one time (Youngson, 1992).

Epidemiological studies measure the association between risk and the
actual disease or infection, enabling interventions to be targeted in order
to change risk behaviour. Taking the example of sexually transmitted
infections, Catchpole (1996) concludes that the control of these infections
depends on the interruption of transmission of infection and the prevention of complications. To achieve this it is important to know which
exposures to infection are risky and what treatments and interventions
are successful in decreasing the risks of exposure. Control measures for

many infections, including those that are sexually transmitted, are put in place based on epidemiological research often before the infection itself is properly understood, e.g. HIV prevention strategies in the mid 1980s. For viral sexually transmitted infections in particular, where no cure is readily available, primary prevention is the only effective control mechanism. Target groups can be identified by epidemiological studies, and control strategies developed accordingly.

Surveillance is also important in order to monitor and audit control programmes. Evaluation of interventions is vital to monitor the effectiveness of existing strategies and catalyse further research.

HISTORY

In 1913 the Royal Commission on Venereal Diseases was established in Britain in response to surveys demonstrating that by 1863 venereal disease accounted for one-third of all sickness in the armed forces (Hall, 1993). As a result, in 1916 a free and confidential service for those with sexually transmitted infections was set up in the United Kingdom. Prior to this there had been no effective or consistent means of recording the incidence of such infections.

Before 1916 the only statistics available were those pertaining to the incidence of syphilis and gonorrhoea and the accuracy of even these was questionable. The figures were collected mainly by the armed forces but were thought to grossly underestimate the real situation. Around 1910 the number of deaths caused by syphilis was unofficially estimated to be 20,000 per year whereas the official figures declared 2000 per year.

In other parts of the world a similar strategy was adopted. In Ontario (in Canada) and Germany commissions were formed and legislation followed on the control of sexually transmitted infections. Specialist clinical services were set up and sexually transmitted infections were included in the list of notifiable diseases in these and many other countries.

Epidemiological research has developed rapidly and new methodologies have improved surveillance of infections, for example, anonymous unlinked testing for HIV. With emphasis switching to the control of viral infections, surveillance systems now need to adapt to provide information as to why the incidence of these infections is changing and how they should be tackled.

THE SITUATION IN THE UNITED KINGDOM

The incidence of sexually transmitted infections in the United Kingdom continues to rise. The reasons for this may be:

- The age of sexual maturity has lowered, therefore many people are having sexual intercourse younger.
- Increased use of the contraceptive pill and intrauterine devices means that fewer barrier methods are used for contraception.
- More sophisticated contact-tracing methods and growing public awareness mean that cases of sexually transmitted infections are recorded more accurately.

METHODS OF CONTROL OF SEXUALLY TRANSMITTED INFECTIONS

Contact tracing

The main control strategy employed by GUM clinics endeavouring to reduce the incidence of sexually transmitted infections is contact tracing. Contact tracing is not a new concept, however, compulsory measures are not considered appropriate and there is no legislation for them. Contact tracing is accepted practice in GUM clinics in the United Kingdom and is considered essential to the management of STIs. The main aims of contact tracing are (Sutton and Payne, 1996):

- to reduce the incidence of reinfection
- to identify and treat contacts of those with sexually transmitted infections
- to prevent further spread of infections
- to prevent the complications of infections left untreated

Effective contact tracing requires excellent communication skills, and training is important. In most GUM clinics, contact tracing is carried out by health advisers although many nurses and some medical personnel are also involved. Whoever is responsible for contact tracing will require the following skills:

- basic counselling skills and excellent communication skills
- in-depth knowledge of the epidemiology of STIs
- awareness of the psychological implications of STIs
- recognition of the importance of confidentiality
- accurate documentation
- recognition of boundaries and when to refer to other sources

The process of contact tracing is ideally begun at the time of diagnosis and consists of an interview with the patient. The following issues will be discussed (Sutton and Payne, 1996):

- modes of transmission of infections
- risks to partners

- the danger of asymptomatic infections
- the danger of reinfection
- risks of complications with untreated infections
- risks to future partners

Contact slips are issued containing confidential codes relating to specific infections and the patient is encouraged to pass these on to their contacts. If and when the contacts attend a GUM clinic they may be given epidemiological treatment or the results of the tests awaited before treatment is administered. This depends upon local policy and the perceived seriousness of the particular condition. In exceptional circumstances when a contact cannot attend, treatment may be given to the index patient to pass on to their contact.

Although contact tracing is well established in GUM clinics, no such control strategy is employed for sexually transmitted infections diagnosed in other centres. In the future, contact tracing could be used by community services, e.g. in GP surgeries and family planning clinics, so as to improve the management of these infections.

The advent of HIV has provoked further discussion on the issue of contact tracing or, to use its more recent title, partner notification. This is discussed further in Chapter 16.

Health education

In order to change behaviour and attitudes, opportunities for patient education must be taken. This can take the form of a display of leaflets in GUM clinics and other health care facilities. Videos and information about support groups are also useful. Nurses should take the opportunity to provide information about safer sex and the use of condoms. Some nurses are trained in family planning and can offer contraceptive advice when appropriate.

Nurses must be skilful in assessing the risks to each individual they see in order to give the most appropriate advice. Cultural and lifestyle differences must be taken into consideration and a non-judgemental attitude adopted. Apparent acceptance of all facets of human sexuality is important in eliciting information and encouraging disclosure in order to achieve open discussion and to maximize opportunities for patient education.

EPIDEMIOLOGY OF SPECIFIC SEXUALLY TRANSMITTED INFECTIONS

Syphilis

The incidence of syphilis varies dramatically around the world and although the advent of penicillin initially had a great impact, in many countries this has not been maintained. Syphilis was a major problem especially during the First World War. In 1918, 27,000 cases were reported in the United Kingdom, rising to 42,000 in 1919. Taking account of the unsophisticated reporting methods of the time, this may be a gross underestimate of the true figure.

In the United Kingdom the incidence of syphilis has declined gradually and remained steady for the past decade (Department of Health, 1995). More men than women continue to be affected, homosexually acquired syphilis contributing to this disparity, although this too is on the decline. In England there were 1393 new cases of syphilis in 1994, 304 of the cases being infectious syphilis. The median age of these individuals was 32 years and 20% of cases were known to be homosexually acquired (Department of Health, 1995).

Due to the control of early syphilis and the screening of all pregnant women for syphilis, congenital syphilis is now rare in developed countries.

Unlike the United Kingdom, the USA has seen a continuous rise in the incidence of primary and secondary syphilis since 1950 (Aral, 1996). This may be due to the mass removal of resources from STI control programmes to HIV and AIDS, as well as due to factors such as poverty. In the UK a similar shift of funding occurred but much of the resources have been used to improve GU services as a whole rather than solely for the funding of HIV services. A rise in incidence has also been reported in the Baltic states and in Russia (Linglof, 1995).

Gonorrhoea

The World Health Organisation (WHO) report approximately 200 million cases of gonorrhoea per year. This is probably a gross underestimate of the problem as many developing countries have no standardized STI control programme and therefore no way of collecting accurate data.

In the United Kingdom gonorrhoea was rife in the early part of this century. In 1918, 17,000 cases were recorded, rising to 38,000 in 1919, again probably an underestimate of the true figure. In England in 1994 the number of new cases of gonorrhoea was the lowest ever recorded, 11,574 (Department of Health, 1995) (see Figure 3.1). This may be due to the safer-sex campaigns to prevent the spread of HIV. The figures for 1994 may be analysed as follows:

By sex: Men – a rate of 46 cases per 100,000
          Women – a rate of 28 cases per 100,000
By age: Men – highest rates in the 16–19, 20–24 and 25–35 age groups
          Women – highest rates in the 16–19 and 20–24 age groups

In the 20–24 age group there has been a recent downward trend for both

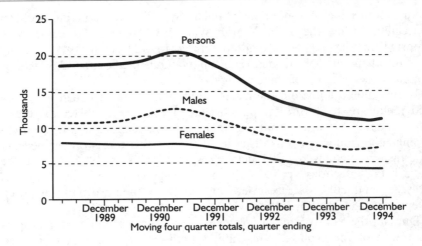

Figure 3.1 New cases of gonorrhoea, England (Department of Health, 1995).

sexes. Homosexually acquired gonorrhoea accounts for 20% of new cases and may be increasing.

Cases of epidemiological treatment contribute an increasing proportion of the total figures for gonorrhoea. This refers to treatment given to contacts of patients known to have gonorrhoea before the diagnosis has been confirmed.

Penicillinase-producing *Neisseria gonorrhoeae* (PPNG)

This resistant strain of gonorrhoea was first discovered in Africa in 1975 and has now been observed in 67 different countries. In the United Kingdom the rise of this strain was mainly due to imported cases but later shifted to indigenous spread. Initially the number of cases doubled at an alarming rate but this strain is now responsible for only 2% of the total incidence of gonorrhoea.

Chlamydia

The annual number of cases of chlamydia in England has remained constant since 1989, around 35,000. It is difficult to ascertain the incidence before then as figures for chlamydia were not reported separately from other sexually transmitted infections. The figures for 1994 may be analysed as follows (Department of Health, 1995):

By sex: Higher incidence in women than men
By age: Most commonly postpubertal

Women – most common in 16–19, 20–24 and 25–34 age groups

Men – most common in 20–24 and 25–34 age groups

Only 2% of cases in 1995 were reported as acquired through homosexual contact. Epidemiological treatment accounted for 23% of the total figures for chlamydia in 1994. This has increased from 15% in 1989.

Pelvic inflammatory disease (PID)

In most countries throughout the world the incidence of PID is on the increase. In England the incidence of PID has steadily risen to 9,214 in 1994. These infections appear to be mainly non-specific but with the largest proportion of identified infection caused by chlamydia. Gonorrhoea is still responsible for a small proportion. Again these figures are probably an underestimate, mainly due to the diagnosis and treatment of PID in centres other than GUM clinics. This highlights the need for improved liaison with other hospital departments, such as gynaecology and accident and emergency, and also with primary health care centres in the community.

This continued rise in cases of PID has many implications for the health of those affected, such as decreased fertility, long-term complications and ectopic pregnancy. Moreover repeated treatment and hospital admissions prove very costly (see Figure 3.2).

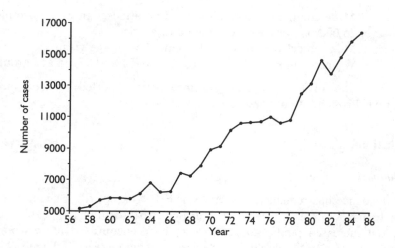

Figure 3.2 Hospital admissions for pelvic inflammatory disease in England and Wales 1958–1981, England only 1982–1985 (Csonka and Oates, 1990).

Herpes simplex (HSV)

The incidence of HSV in England has steadily increased since 1988 to 26,800 in 1994. This includes both primary and recurrent attacks. Recurrent attacks account for 43% of the total. The figures may be analysed as follows (Department of Health, 1995) (see Figure 3.3):

By sex: Women account for 59% of first-attack cases
          In men the incidence has remained quite stable
By age: Men – highest incidence in 20–24, 25–34 and 35–44 age groups
          Women – highest incidence in 16–19, 20–24 and 25–34 age groups

In 1994 5% of cases were reported as acquired through homosexual contact. In the USA there is no standard method of data collection for genital herpes but it is estimated that between 2 and 20 million people are affected.

Genital warts

There has been a slow upward trend in the incidence of genital warts in England since the late 1980s, reaching a figure of 86,700 in 1994. Recurrent attacks accounted for 43% of the total. The rise has been due to the increased incidence of recurrent attacks, the number of first attacks having remained steady since these figures were first reported separately in 1989. The figures may be analysed as follows (Department of Health, 1995) (see Figure 3.3):

By sex: More common in men although first attack figures are around 25,000 per year for both men and women
By age: Men – most common in 20–24 and 25–34 age groups
          Women – most common in 16–19, 20–24 and 25–34 age groups

Five per cent of the new cases in men were reported to have been acquired through homosexual contact.

Vaginal infections

Candidiasis

The incidence has remained constant since 1984 except for a slight rise in 1994 to 64,787 cases per year. It is difficult to ascertain the reasons for this, but increased public awareness may have encouraged more women to present at GUM clinics for diagnosis. The increased diagnosis of candida may be incidental to women attending clinics for other reasons, such as colposcopy.

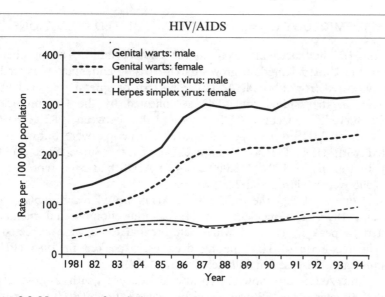

Figure 3.3 New cases of genital warts and genital infection with HSV seen in GUM clinics (combined first attack and recurrent infection), 1981–1994. Source: *Communicable Disease Report*, Vol 5, No. 39, 29 September 1995. Reproduced with permission of the PHLS Communicable Disease Surveillance Centre © PHLS.

Trichomoniasis

The incidence has greatly decreased in England, to 5559 cases per year in 1994. This may be connected with the fall in incidence of gonorrhoea, for these two infections were often linked.

Anaerobic vaginosis

Since cases began to be reported separately in 1989 the incidence has risen to 53,894 in 1994. Again a reason for this may be the increased number of women presenting at GUM clinics.

Hepatitis B

The number of new cases of hepatitis B in England in 1994 was 471 and has remained steady since 1989 (Department of Health, 1995). Seventy-five per cent of these cases are males, one-third of the infections being acquired through homosexual contact.

Cases of other kinds of viral hepatitis had trebled by 1994, probably due to the increased testing for hepatitis C.

HIV/AIDS

HIV is a relatively new infection; it was only recently, in 1985 that the first person died of AIDS in a London hospital. At this time over 300 cases of HIV had been identified in the United States. The number of cases in the United Kingdom grew quickly, arising endemically as well as being imported from abroad. A similar pattern of spread was evident to that seen in the United States. Data collected by the Communicable Disease Surveillance Centre (CDSC) showed that between 1982 and 1994, 9436 cases of AIDS were reported and 22,000 people were known to be infected with HIV (PHLS Communicable Disease Surveillance Centre, 1994). In Europe by 1994, 118,000 cases of AIDS had been reported. Of these 4505 were children and 2250 women.

It was predicted that the incidence of AIDS would reach a plateau in 1996 and 1997. The incidence of HIV among homosexual men was expected to peak in 1993–94 while heterosexual cases were expected to rise. The incidence of HIV among drug users peaked in 1985 (PHLS Communicable Disease Surveillance Centre, 1993).

HIV and AIDS are now a worldwide concern, with almost every country affected. The World Health Organisation (WHO) reported 851,628 cases of AIDS worldwide by 1994. The real figure is probably close to three million. The WHO predictions for the year 2000 are 8–24 million cases of AIDS in adults. An additional 30–40 million people may be infected with HIV (WHO, 1993).

REPORTING OF SEXUALLY TRANSMITTED INFECTIONS

There is a well established system for the reporting of sexually transmitted infections in the United Kingdom. Every GUM clinic in England is required to submit quarterly returns on a KC60 form (described in more detail later in this chapter). This enables more accurate data to be generated, and informed decisions made in targeting the resourcing of prevention programmes.

It is important to recognize that many of the data reflect only those attending GUM clinics; underreporting is a problem in many countries including the United Kingdom. There are several reasons for underreporting:

1. Some STIs are diagnosed and treated outside GUM clinics, e.g. GP surgeries, family planning clinics and other departments within hospitals. These go unreported in many cases.
2. Some people may have STIs without realising and these may be inadvertently treated with antibiotics intended for another purpose.
3. There may be differences in the way data are collected in each clinic, which may cause inconsistencies.
4. Private medical consultations for diagnosis and treatment of sexually transmitted infections may go unreported.

STATISTICAL RETURNS

The workload of GUM clinics is monitored by the analysis of two main sources of statistical (Korner) data provided by each GUM clinic. These data form the basis for determining the national incidence of sexually transmitted infections. Two types of information are collected, information pertaining to the number of diagnoses in each clinic and information about the workload of each clinic.

KC60

This is a quarterly return that provides information on the number of different diagnoses seen in GUM clinics. These figures will differ from the attendance figures as one person may have several different diagnoses.

The KC60 is a confidential document that records all diagnoses as codes without disclosing any personal information. The information required on this form has recently changed to include many new diagnoses, e.g. pre-test counselling for HIV.

From these returns it is possible to view data broken down according to:

- gender
- age
- infections acquired homosexually

It is inevitable that with so many different people entering data on the KC60 returns, inconsistencies are common, but these documents do give a useful national picture of the incidence and prevalence of sexually transmitted infections including HIV and AIDS.

KH09

This is completed on a monthly basis and records the number of clinic sessions held and the number of patient visits to the GUM clinic. This report contains the following data:

- number of clinic sessions held
- number of clinic sessions cancelled
- number of referrals seen (new or rebooked patients, i.e. those attending with a new condition or new episode)
- number of referrals who did not attend
- number of consultant-initiated attendances seen (follow-up)
- number of consultant-initiated attendances who did not attend
- number of GP referrals
- number of private patient attendances
- number of contractual arrangement attendances

The last two do not apply at present to GUM clinics but to general outpatients.

There are many problems with the consistency of these returns. These include:

- Variation in the definition of a clinic session.
- Confusion as to whether bank holidays should be recorded as cancelled clinic sessions.
- Some patients are not recorded if they saw a nurse or health adviser but not a doctor.
- It is difficult to record patients who did not attend if the clinic provides a walk-in service.
- Confusion regarding the recording of telephone calls.
- Clinics without computer systems have difficulty in collecting data.

SUMMARY

A comprehensive network of GU services in the United Kingdom did well to control the spread of gonorrhoea and syphilis in the first half of this century and in expanding to deal with other aspects of sexual health. Recent trends show that the bacterial sexually transmitted infections are in general decreasing. Unfortunately in recent years the incidence of viral infections has increased dramatically and these have proved more challenging to diagnose and treat. In addition many of these infections, such as HIV, hepatitis B and hepatitis C, have more serious consequences for the individual affected and their contacts. They often have longer incubation periods, making contact tracing more difficult, and in many cases cannot be satisfactorily treated.

As new drugs and methods of treatment are developed it will be interesting to observe the trends in sexually transmitted viral infections and the effect these will continue to have on the structure and scope of GU services.

Systems for reporting sexually transmitted infections vary from country to country and should only be compared with caution. In many countries the incidence of STIs is grossly underestimated, and hence prevention and health education programmes are underresourced. The reporting of the incidence of sexually transmitted infections is less accurate in the USA, where many people are treated in private clinics not required to report to a national body. In many developing countries the reporting systems are unsophisticated and inconsistent, resulting in gross underestimation of the incidence of sexually transmitted infections. Accurate epidemiological studies are essential in order to mobilize funding and political support for public health strategies for the control of these infections. Such studies can also demonstrate the cost-effectiveness of control programmes.

REFERENCES

Aral, S.O. (1996) The social context of syphilis persistence in the south-eastern United States. *Sexually Transmitted Diseases*, **23**(1), 9–15.

Catchpole, M.A. (1996) The role of epidemiology and surveillance systems in the control of sexually transmitted diseases. *Genitourinary Medicine*, **72**(5), 321–9.

Csonka, G.W. and Oates, J.K. (1990) *Sexually Transmitted Diseases: A Textbook of Genitourinary Medicine*, Baillière Tindall, London.

Department of Health (1995) *Statistical Bulletin: Sexually Transmitted Diseases, England 1994*, Bulletin 1995/16.

Hall, L.A. (1993) 'The Cinderella of Medicine': sexually-transmitted diseases in Britain in the nineteenth and twentieth centuries. *Genitourinary Medicine*, **69**(3) 314–19.

Linglof, T. (1995) Rapid increase of syphilis and gonorrhoea in parts of the former USSR. *Sexually Transmitted Diseases*, **22**(3), 160–1.

Meers, P., Sedgwick, J. and Worsley, M. (1995) *The Microbiology and Epidemiology of Infection for Health Science Students*, Chapman & Hall, London.

PHLS Communicable Disease Surveillance Centre (1993) The incidence and prevalence of AIDS and other severe HIV disease in England and Wales for 1992–1997: projections using data to the end of June 1992. *Communicable Disease Report*, **3**(Suppl.1), S1–S17.

PHLS Communicable Disease Surveillance Centre (1994) AIDS and HIV infection in the United Kingdom: monthly report. *Communicable Disease Report*, **4**(28), 131–4.

Sutton, A. and Payne, S. (1996) *Genito-urinary Medicine for Nurses*, Whurr, London.

WHO (1993) Press release, WHO/69 (7 September). World Health Organisation, Geneva.

Youngson, R.M. (1992) *Collins Dictionary of Medicine*, HarperCollins, Glasgow.

4

Psychological aspects of genitourinary medicine

Jenny Wilks

OBJECTIVES

1. To recognise the psychological and emotional issues that can affect people attending GUM clinics.
2. To describe the psychological sequelae of sexually transmitted infections, particularly the impact of HIV infection.
3. To summarize additional psychological concerns that are likely to present at GUM clinics.
4. To recognise the importance of taking psychological factors into account, for adequate treatment and prevention of sexually transmitted infections.
5. To explain the role of counselling in GUM clinics and the nurse's contribution to this.

INTRODUCTION

The interface between illness and sexuality gives the field of genitourinary medicine a particular range of emotional and psychological implications. Before a person even attends a GUM clinic, they must have been through a decision-making process – either alone or in consultation with their GP – which has led them to believe that they have been at risk of contracting an infection. Clinic users often arrive with high levels of anxiety and with negative preconceptions about the GUM service (Evans and Farquhar, 1996). Staff, who have seen it all before, can all too easily forget that patients may be completely unfamiliar with the clinic setting and unaware of the examination and treatment procedures that will be followed.

Historically GU medicine has been a 'basement speciality', tucked away at the back of the hospital. This facilitates anonymity, but it may reflect and reinforce people's shame about the stigma that is still attached to attendance at such a clinic. Genitourinary medicine staff may wish to reduce the stigma and to site their clinics closer to other hospital departments. However, Munday (1990) found that patients stated a preference for the GUM clinic to be sited away from the main outpatients department. If we do not take this preference into account we may lose patients' trust and collaboration. Similar considerations apply with regard to confidentiality: most patients do not want their GP to know about their clinic attendance. A balance needs to be found between assuring confidentiality while encouraging people to bring their contacts in for treatment. Since successful treatment prevents the development of late complications of sexually transmitted infections, it is important to try to meet clients' needs and preferences. The more that GUM staff can put people at their ease, the more likely it is they will keep future appointments, which is important in assessing the efficacy of treatment.

PSYCHOLOGICAL ISSUES IN GU MEDICINE

In addition to these general psychological considerations, some GUM patients have particular psychological difficulties. Until the mid 1980s, it was relatively rare for psychological issues to be seriously addressed in the GUM setting. No clinical psychologists were employed specifically in this field and the role of health advisers was largely restricted to contact tracing. This began to change because GUM clinics became the main location of treatment for HIV infection, and the psychological and emotional issues needs of people with HIV became obvious. In time the demand became such that specialist clinical psychologists were employed in this area and the role of the health adviser was broadened to include more counselling, especially in relation to the HIV antibody test that was introduced in 1985. One effect of this development has been the identification of, and response to, a previously untapped and unmet need for psychological help among GUM clinic attenders other than those affected by HIV and AIDS. Although much has been written about psychological aspects of HIV and AIDS (eg. Green and McCreaner, 1996), less attention has been given to other aspects of psychological care in this field.

There are several reasons why GUM clinic attenders may need psychological help. Most (though not all) of the conditions for which people are treated at GUM clinics are sexually transmitted and this raises several issues that may lead to psychological difficulties, including the social stigma of STIs and their implications for sexual relationships. Some genitourinary infections, notably herpes, are not curable and this raises similar psychological issues as for coping with any other chronic health problem. In the setting of a GUM clinic, when people are discussing sexual issues and being examined intimately, they may also feel able to mention problems they might not have felt comfortable to raise with their GP, for example psychosexual difficulties, or issues relating to past sexual abuse or assault.

The problems presented generally fall into the following categories, although problem areas often overlap and more than one category may apply in any particular case.

Psychological aspects of sexually acquired infections

To some extent all illnesses involve psychological and social aspects as well as physical conditions. The diagnostic label influences both the behaviour of the person affected and the attitudes and actions of others – including society at large – toward the 'patient'. However, illnesses vary greatly in the extent to which this has an impact on the person diagnosed, depending on factors such as: mortality, disfigurement, contagiousness and infectiousness (perceived or actual), sexual overtones, mental effects, and the social groups that are most affected. Thus, at one extreme, vaginal thrush (unless it is HIV related) is unlikely to have major psychological sequelae, because few of the above factors pertain. At the other extreme, in HIV disease all these factors operate to some extent and this affects both other people's reactions and the emotional response of the person diagnosed. A major influence on personal and social attitudes to all STIs is the fact that they are often seen as evidence of a particular kind of sexual lifestyle (so-called 'promiscuity') even though this may or may not be so in an individual situation, and is in any case irrelevant to medical treatment.

The emotional and psychological difficulties following a diagnosis of any illness are of two broad kinds. Firstly there is the direct result of the diagnosis and all its implications. Secondly there may be a renewed experience of prior psychological problems or restimulation of previous traumatic events, which can complicate the response to the diagnosis. People diagnosed with STIs and other genitourinary infections may have problems coping with both the medical condition and the effects on their life and relationships. They may experience feelings such as guilt, anxiety, depression and loss of self-esteem. Similar psychological issues are involved in all sexually transmitted infections – the specific diagnosis is crucial for medical purposes but is often not the most important factor influencing psychological response. However, HIV is of course a particular case because of its seriousness, and it will therefore be considered separately.

Before the advent of HIV, the most feared STI was probably genital herpes, because there is as yet no cure. It has faded from the public eye, but its prevalence continues to rise. Treatment of herpes has been greatly enhanced in the last decade or so by the availability of antiviral agents, especially acyclovir. For people with frequently recurring herpes, suppressive acyclovir treatment has been shown to reduce the psychological and psychosexual problems associated with their condition (Carney *et al.*, 1993).

However, the psychological effects of herpes can be more problematic and long-lasting than the physical symptoms. Even if someone does not experience recurrent attacks, the knowledge that they are still carrying the herpes virus can profoundly change their self-image. After diagnosis they have to acknowledge their new identity as a 'person with herpes'. They may have had ideas about what sort of person contracts such an infection, and have to adapt to being such a person themselves. Because herpes carries connotations of promiscuity and incurability, the new identity adopted is likely to be a negative one and may be accompanied by disbelief, fear, isolation, helplessness, frustration and depression (Helsen and Kinghorn, 1991).

For most people, the area of life most affected by a diagnosis of herpes is of course that of sexual relationships. For people who have a regular partner, there is the problem of how to tell their partner their diagnosis and the fear they may be rejected if they do so. If the partner also has herpes, they may feel they cannot leave the relationship even if it is unsatisfactory, because of the fear that they will not be able to find another partner. For those without a regular partner, the diagnosis has implications when they meet prospective partners, of whether to tell them and when. For women planning to have a child there is anxiety about the risk to the baby.

There is evidence that psychological factors including emotional stress can be important in triggering the recurrence of genital herpes. Dalkvist and colleagues (1995) found that recurrences of genital herpes were preceded by reduced overall emotional well-being over a ten-day period. Swanson, Dibble and Chenitz (1995) report that young adults with herpes perceived stress to be the major cause of recurrent attacks. This can be a vicious cycle, since recurrent attacks, or worry about the possibility of them, can themselves be very stressful. Learning to manage and cope with the stresses caused by herpes can therefore have a significant effect not only on emotional well-being but on the process of the disease itself.

Drob, Loemer and Lifshutz (1985) describe the impact of herpes on the lives of 42 people. Nearly all reported a profound effect on sexual behaviour and on interpersonal relationships in general. Emotional responses, especially depression and anger, were common, as was reduced self-confidence. They also suggest that the negative consequences of herpes can sometimes take on the psychological function of providing an excuse for retreat from the effort of establishing adult relationships and interpersonal intimacy where these were already problematic areas. Those most vulnerable to a severe psychological reaction to herpes are therefore likely to be those whose self-esteem was fragile prior to diagnosis. This complicates psychological therapy, since the person's reaction to herpes is unlikely to change until they can find ways to resolve the broader issue.

However Drob, Loemer and Lifshutz also stress that for most people with herpes, recurrences are infrequent and excellent adjustment is likely. Indeed, some of their subjects reported that their diagnosis gave them the impetus to examine their lives and make positive changes, including 'a refocusing upon non-sexual aspects of friendship and intimacy in their relationships, greater attention to their general health, and a better understanding and tolerance of the problems of others'.

Even in those STIs that can be successfully treated, there may be psychological ramifications which persist when the infection has been eradicated. Faxelid and Krantz (1993) report self-blame among most patients with chlamydia and found that the diagnosis had led to fear of HIV among a significant proportion. Stronks and colleagues (1993) compared the psychological consequences of herpes and gonorrhoea and found little difference between the two groups of patients. However, those with herpes judged themselves to have had fewer psychological complaints prior to the disease, which suggests they were more inclined to perceive their current complaints as a direct result of their condition than were the gonorrhoea patients.

One of the most frequently seen problems in GUM clinics is infection with genital warts, caused by the human papillomavirus (HPV). With such a common condition, there is perhaps more risk of staff underestimating the emotional effects on the patient. Voog and Lowhagen (1992) point out that genital warts can be a long-lasting and relapsing condition, and that this, along with the association of the virus with cancer, puts much stress on the person affected. Chandler (1996) reported high levels of anxiety in women with warts at their first clinic attendance, as well as much uncertainty about the methods of treatment. Filiberti and colleagues (1993), studying patients with widespread wart virus infection, found significant levels of self-blame, sexual and relationship difficulties, and fear of cancer.

Women with cervical HPV infection and other abnormal smears may be referred for colposcopy, which may further increase their anxiety. Bennetts and colleagues (1995), using factor analysis of questionnaire data, identified four dimensions of distress in women undergoing colposcopy: prior experience of medical procedures, beliefs/feelings about cervical abnormality and changes in perception of oneself, worry about infectivity, and the effect on sexual relationships. Tomaino-

Brunner, Freda and Runowicz (1996) found that women referred for colposcopy were anxious about their health, uncertain about the meaning of their cervical smear results and apprehensive and ill-informed about colposcopy. They recommend longer appointment time to provide appropriate education and to help alleviate women's anxiety. Although cervical screening is known to be effective in reducing the incidence of cancer, these psychological costs need to be taken into account. Bell and colleagues (1995) found that for women undergoing cytological surveillance following mild or moderate dyskaryotic smears, their level of anxiety was related to their degree of satisfaction with the explanation provided. Health care staff need to be careful to check with patients whether they have received, and understood, the information they need. Marteau and colleagues (1996) compared two information booklets that were sent out with appointment letters. They found that giving complex information only increased knowledge without affecting anxiety. A booklet that was more simply written and included strategies for coping as well as basic information was more effective in reducing anxiety about colposcopy.

HIV/AIDS

Infection with the human immunodeficiency virus (HIV), along with its clinical consequence of AIDS, occupies a unique position in GUM because it is both incurable and life threatening. Additionally, it is a relatively new condition (having been first identified in 1981), and medical opinion and treatment options are rapidly changing. People presenting with psychological problems related to HIV/AIDS include not only people with HIV, but also their partners and relatives and people who have been bereaved through AIDS. These are of course not mutually exclusive categories. Members of the communities most affected by HIV (gay men, people from sub-Saharan Africa and intravenous drug users) are often part of a social network that includes many other people who are HIV positive. This can be a source of support: people feel that they are not alone with their diagnosis. But it also means that many people with HIV have already suffered bereavements because of the virus and this influences both their reaction to other people's illness and their ability to deal with HIV themselves.

The long-term process of coming to terms with, and learning to live with, HIV may begin even before being tested. If the person has initiated the request for testing, they have already had reason to suspect they are positive and will have spent time considering the implications of a positive result. Others, however, have not even considered the possibility of HIV infection until they become unwell; the test may then be recommended by a doctor and the patient has not had the opportunity to do this anticipatory work. In either case, it is crucial that they receive adequate counselling before being tested. The quality of the whole experience of being tested can affect long-term coping ability.

Even with satisfactory pre-test and post-test counselling, there is no typical response to a diagnosis of HIV or AIDS. For example, someone who has the test because they are aware of prior risky behaviour, has thought through the implications of the test and wants to know their status, will have a different experience from someone who has the test in a state of shock because they have just found out that their partner has AIDS. The context in which a positive result occurs (in other words the individual's life history and current situation) will influence the impact of the result. This context is unique for each person and includes factors such as:

- prior experience and understanding of HIV and AIDS
- severity of symptoms of illness (if any)
- personal, social and financial resources
- attitude of family, friends and partner
- previous experience of illness
- general coping skills and psychological health
- feelings about the behaviour that led to infection
- the reason they were tested and how they were told the result

However, common themes in the reaction to discovering that one is HIV positive include the following:

Shock

Both when someone is first tested and whenever there is any major change or deterioration in their condition, they are likely to have a period of being in shock emotionally. This may be evidenced by denial, extreme emotional upset, and confusion. However, even when a person appears calm on the surface they may be in shock and in this state may not really take in what health care staff say to them about their condition and its treatment.

Anger

People may be angry with the person who infected them (if known), though more commonly there is a less specific anger towards the situation that led to them becoming HIV positive. This may include self-blame and feelings of resentment towards people who are not infected. Anger may be directed at health care staff, especially the 'bearers of bad news'. It is important for workers to be able to acknowledge this anger and not take it personally.

Uncertainty

This is perhaps the most ubiquitous theme in living with HIV. It affects people at all points on the continuum of HIV disease. People experience much uncertainty about future prognosis, illnesses they may suffer, treatment they may be offered and its efficacy, when and how they will die and whether there will be any major treatment breakthroughs in time to benefit them. They may also be uncertain about how significant others will cope and about how their condition will affect their work, social life and so on. This experience of not knowing often feels worse than receiving clear information, even if it is bad news. Health care staff may be tempted to allay uncertainty by trying to give clear advice and prognosis, but this is impossible to do accurately. In particular, it is not helpful to talk in terms of how many months or years a person might live, since this can rarely be predicted with any precision.

Anxiety

This is closely related to the above uncertainties. People with HIV often experience understandable fear about the future, especially about pain, illness and death – often not so much of death *per se* but of dying in pain, or of being left alone when they are ill or dying because others cannot cope.

Depression

People with HIV often feel helpless, hopeless about the future and out of control of their lives. They may experience self-recrimination about the whole situation. People often feel that the virus is in charge of their lives and that their autonomy is eroded by the demands of medical treatment. Also their decline in health eventually places limitations on their social and work activities, reducing their quality of life. This may be exacerbated by the experience of bereavement or other losses. All of these factors can lead to depression.

Loss of self-esteem

Although at a conscious, rational level people may reject societal prejudice and hostility towards people with HIV, this can be internalized at a more unconscious level. It is difficult to maintain high self-esteem knowing that you have such a stigmatized illness, especially if you have experienced rejection or negative responses from others, or if you are keeping it secret for fear of this. Self-esteem can also be damaged if HIV disease leads to visible deterioration in appearance, for example extreme weight loss or disfigurement.

The prevalence and severity of these issues varies widely between individuals and for an individual through time. Each new change in health status may exacerbate emotional difficulties. The long-term process of living with HIV tends to go in cycles: the person may come to some degree of reconciliation with one aspect of their condition (e.g. the positive result) and for a while they cope well. But during the course of HIV disease various changes occur which may re-evoke the same kinds of responses as did the original test result. Such changes include:

- progression from asymptomatic to symptomatic illness
- a significant drop in CD4 count or increase in viral load
- starting treatment (or being advised to do so by doctors)
- deciding to enter experimental drug trials
- telling family or significant others
- entering a new relationship
- partner or friends developing HIV-related illness
- pregnancy
- stopping work for health reasons

Responses to any of the above will also be influenced by the same mediating factors as affected response to the initial diagnosis of HIV, though some of these may have changed in the interim.

The psychological sequelae of HIV and AIDS are complicated by the possibility of neurological damage. Where this is caused by an opportunistic infection (e.g. cerebral toxoplasmosis) accurate diagnosis is essential as this may be treatable. However, HIV itself can affect the central nervous system, and the effects of this can include apparent emotional problems, e.g. poor concentration, confusion, apathy, and mood or personality changes. Conversely, stress and anxiety can mimic or mask neurological abnormalities. Psychometric testing and CAT/MRI scans are essential to clarify diagnosis where there are suspected neurological changes. However, it is not always possible to tease out the relative contributions of physical and psychological reasons for cognitive difficulties. In either case, counselling needs to take account of limitations imposed by cognitive changes, but in such a way that the patient retains as much control as possible over what is happening. When patients are slow to understand, there is a danger that professionals take over decision making, which will increase the person's confusion and distress. The aim is more that their cognitive vulnerability should be recognized and allowed for (Kocsis, 1996).

Psychological therapy for people with HIV/AIDS

Despite the above range of possible difficulties, not all people with HIV or AIDS will need or want to be referred to specialist counsellors or psychologists. Much informal counselling and support takes place during interactions with nurses and other staff when people attend the clinic.

The general aims of counselling in this area include:

- giving structure to what can feel like an overwhelming situation, in order to make problem areas more manageable and to help the person address 'dreaded issues' (Bor and Miller, 1988);
- helping the person to regain some control of their lives;
- creating a safe and confidential relationship in which topics can be addressed which may be taboo in most or all other relationships;
- utilizing specific therapeutic interventions to help people deal with particular difficulties, for example anxiety management or cognitive/ behavioural therapy for depression (these are likely to require referral to a counsellor or clinical psychologist).

Counselling in this field is likely to include some discussion of factual information, for example about new treatments that someone may be considering. Liaison among the members of the multidisciplinary team is crucial, to ensure that information is imparted in a way that is consistent and enables people to make informed decisions that will influence their behaviour. Counsellors and other health care staff also need some understanding of the different cultures and lifestyles of the clients they see, and a non-judgemental approach to these. Confidentiality is vital and where information is shared within a team this needs to be clear to the client – often in the NHS information is passed between various staff members without patients being aware of how many people have access to it. This is important in all areas of health, but any breaches of confidentiality can have particularly serious social consequences for people with HIV/ AIDS.

Counselling with HIV-positive people often (though not always) touches on areas not often covered in general counselling settings, ranging from details of sexual practices to planning funerals. Counselling is one of the few socially sanctioned relationships where intimate behaviour and existential questions can be openly and confidentially discussed; and an effective counsellor must not be judgemental or embarrassed. All staff in this field should be comfortable talking about any topic that might come up, since there may be nowhere else in the person's life that certain issues can be raised.

Problems related to sexual behaviour

Many people attending GUM clinics are experiencing problems in sexual relationships (heterosexual or homosexual). For some patients, the diagnosis of an STI leads to relationship difficulties because it is the first inkling they have of their partner's infidelity. This leads to a double blow.

Not only have they to cope with being told that they have contracted a sexually transmitted infection, but they have to deal with the implicit message that their partner may not have been faithful. Sometimes of course this suspicion may be unfounded – the infection pre-dates the relationship but had never been diagnosed. This is particularly likely in conditions that do not necessarily have symptoms. However, this can still lead to mistrust and affect the relationship. A particular difficulty for staff occurs when someone is saying one thing to their partner and something else to staff. We have to respond to this appropriately without breaching confidentiality.

Even when psychosexual problems are not directly related to an STI, they are often raised in GUM because this is a setting where issues around sexuality are explicitly the focus of attention. The tight standards of confidentiality and anonymity in GUM clinics may help people to feel safe to disclose that they are having sexual difficulties. Gordon (1987) reviews several studies that found a high prevalence of reported psychosexual problems (e.g. lack of arousal or desire, problems reaching orgasm, or pain on intercourse) in GUM clinic attenders, many of whom said that they would have liked further help with these problems. Catalan and colleagues (1981) found that, although patients who were given an STI diagnosis were no less likely than others to have sexual or other psychological problems, medical staff were more likely to comment in the notes on the presence of psychological disturbance or sexual problems when no diagnosis was given. This suggests that when no physical disorder is found, doctors are more likely to explain the patient's attendance and symptoms in psychological terms. Conversely, therefore, psychological and sexual difficulties may be more likely to be missed when patients are found to have an STI: these patients should also be asked about the presence of non-medical difficulties. Sometimes all they may need is some information and reassurance, but in general, people with psychosexual difficulties need to be referred for specialist help. They should first be assessed by medical staff to ensure that there is no organic cause for the problem.

Effects of rape and sexual assault or abuse

Problems related to coercive and/or violent sexual experiences may also be raised in the GUM setting. People may present immediately following a sexual assault, for a check-up, since there is a significant risk of acquiring a sexually transmitted disease as a result of rape (Glaser, Hammerschlag and McCormack, 1989). But many other attenders may have been assaulted some time previously and may mention this during the consultation. People who have been sexually assaulted or abused in the past are significantly more likely to have psychosexual problems (Zverina *et al.*,

1987). They may find it difficult to undergo intimate medical examination. Sensitive questioning by health care staff can ascertain whether someone has a history of sexual trauma, and whether they would like some psychotherapeutic help with the effects of this, however long ago it was. The traumatic effects of sexual assault or abuse can last for a long time, and people carry an additional psychological burden if they have not told anyone about it.

Cahill, Llewelyn and Pearson (1991) review several studies reporting the long-term effects of childhood sexual abuse. These include emotional reactions and self-perceptions such as depression, low self-esteem, distorted beliefs, a sense of being branded or stigmatized, and a great deal of guilt, anger and self-blame. People are also more likely to experience sexual difficulties and relationship problems, such as inability to trust and revictimization, including domestic violence and further non-consensual sexual relationships. There is also some evidence (Arnold *et al.*, 1990) that survivors of childhood sexual abuse may be more vulnerable to physical symptoms, e.g. pelvic pain, which may also lead them to present in a GUM clinic.

Burgess and Holmstrom (1974) describe a constellation of symptoms that may result from rape or sexual assault. This 'rape trauma syndrome' can be seen as a specific type of post-traumatic stress disorder, and includes behavioural, somatic and psychological reactions. Based on interviews with women attending an emergency ward after having been raped, they describe the syndrome as falling into two phases. In the acute phase, immediately after the attack, women experience somatic complaints, fear and self-blame, and a disruption of their lifestyle. At this time, some people express their emotional reactions very openly and are visibly distressed and tearful. Others have a more controlled style of response, appearing quite calm, but they may be in no less a state of shock and staff need to be alert to this. In the second phase the long-term process of reorganization begins, although people may continue to experience the 'acute' symptoms. Other writers, e.g. Bassuk (1980), separate the longer-term response into two stages. The first of these, the recoil phase, involves the implementation of coping mechanisms that lead to a decrease in symptoms and a gradual resumption of normal functioning. However, at this point the traumatic impact of the rape has not been resolved and the woman is going through the motions of normal life. It is in the third reconstitutive phase that she begins to deal with the specific personal meaning she attaches to the rape. Her particular concerns and response will be influenced by previously existing conflicts and life-stage issues. Both models stress that fully re-establishing one's lifestyle and sense of control in the world can take months or years.

These studies, like most research on rape, focused on women. However, GUM staff need to be alert to the even more hidden problem of sexual assault on men, which until recently was barely even recognized. Hillman and colleagues (1990) report on five cases of male victims of assault who presented at GUM clinics. They point out that GUM departments are well placed to meet these men's medical and counselling requirements; however, the environment needs to be supportive and sympathetic to allow men who have been sexually assaulted to overcome their anxiety and ask for help. The taboo on disclosing rape may be greater for men than for women, though for both sexes there are societal attitudes and myths (such as that only 'loose women' are raped or that 'real men' could not be raped) which may compound people's difficulties in accessing support.

People's ability to cope and their need for counselling depend on factors such as the time that has elapsed since the assault, their social support network and whether they have a history of additional psychological or social problems. Where someone has been functioning adequately prior to the assault, short-term crisis-oriented counselling is likely to be sufficient to help them to mobilize their own coping resources. Where other issues arise that require a more in-depth therapeutic response, referral to a more specialist counsellor or psychotherapist is indicated. According to Koss (1993), effective counselling in this area needs to include the avoidance of victim blame, a supportive, non-stigmatizing view of rape, an environment in which to overcome cognitive and behavioural avoidance, information about trauma reactions and the expectation that symptoms will improve.

Problems with safer sex

Another area in which sexual relationships may be problematic is that of putting safer sex guidelines into practice to avoid infection (especially in relation to HIV). It is important not to respond with judgemental or critical comments when people admit to unsafe sex, as this will make them likely to keep quiet about it and prevent them from accessing help. GUM staff have an important role in the prevention of STIs and HIV, but need to be aware that information alone does not necessarily lead to behaviour change. Fishbein and Ajzen's (1975) theory of reasoned action suggests that effective behaviour change depends on other factors, such as whether people believe that such action will lead to desired consequences and whether they think that behaviour change is considered desirable by people whose views matter to them. Consistent with this, Beaman and Strader (1989) found that condom use among GUM patients did not correlate with knowledge about AIDS, but was influenced by beliefs about sexual partners' attitudes towards condoms.

Even when people do want to change their sexual behaviour, this is like changing any longstanding habit – the desire to change may by itself not be enough. They may need therapeutic help in maintaining safer sex and avoiding relapse. Roffman, Gordon and Craver (1987) have developed an approach to relapse prevention that draws on ideas developed in the field of addictive behaviours. The focus is on helping people to develop specific skills for coping with high-risk situations and moods that would otherwise lead to unsafe sex, as well as to develop more satisfying lives and relationships in order to reduce vulnerability to relapsing back into unsafe sexual behaviour.

Anxiety states

Not everyone who attends a GUM clinic is found to have an infection. For most, negative test results offer immediate relief of anxiety, but some people continue to experience severe anxiety despite low risk factors and/ or negative test results. If people are experiencing physical symptoms, and their STI screening is negative, their anxiety about their symptoms may increase rather than decrease. They may fear that they are suffering from a serious illness and are not necessarily reassured by the fact that no medical cause can be found. Fitzpatrick, Frost and Ikkkos (1986) found that 40% of STI clinic attenders had life disruption associated with concern about serious illness. This is particularly common in relation to HIV infection, where this group of people is often termed the 'worried well'.

The worried well often present with anxiety-based symptoms (such as sweating, diarrhoea and fatigue) which they have misinterpreted as evidence of HIV disease. This can be reinforced if their symptoms resemble descriptions of AIDS that they have encountered in the mass media. They may have anxious ruminations about past and present behaviour that they think might have put them at risk (often some activity for which they feel guilt or shame) and about the consequences for themselves and their loved ones if they had HIV. They tend to attend selectively to any information that is consistent with their belief that they have HIV and to ignore or discount contradictory evidence. Although these patients comprise a small proportion of clinic attenders, they can take up an inordinate amount of clinic time. They often tax the sympathy of clinic staff, who are used to working with people who really are physically ill, but it is important to acknowledge the very severe distress that they are experiencing.

The worried well are usually offered repeated testing and continual reassurance, but the effect of this on reducing anxiety is very short-lived. More helpful approaches to this problem are based on seeing it more as a type of hypochondriasis or health preoccupation, which happens to be focused on HIV. Miller, Acton and Hedge (1988) report successful results using a behaviourally based psychotherapeutic approach to the problem, involving strict behavioural contracting, re-interpretation of the causes of the patient's stress, response prevention to modify their behavioural response to that stress, and work on self-esteem. This paradigm is based on the notion that reassurance actually maintains the problematic fears and behaviours, serving much the same purpose (short-term reduction in anxiety) as do rituals in obsessive/compulsive disorders. The effect of this is to contribute to higher levels of anxiety in the longer term and to lead to further seeking of reassurance, which reinforces the person's avoidance of tackling their underlying difficulties. Instead, people need to be helped to change their attributions regarding the causes of their difficulties and to change their behavioural response accordingly. The therapist needs to take the patient's experience and fears seriously, in order to gain their trust, but discussion of the feared illness (usually HIV) should be restricted to a few minutes at the end of the session. The focus is instead on encouraging the person to gather and test evidence that their physical symptoms are based on anxiety rather than illness and to try out strategies other than continued reassurance seeking.

Compliance

Many illnesses require behavioural changes by patients if they are to be treated effectively, and STIs are no exception. At the very least, they need to take prescribed medication as instructed. However, there is evidence that, in all areas of medicine, patients often do not follow instructions for treatment. This is generally labelled 'non-compliance', implying that it is completely the patient's responsibility. However, psychological explanations view the patient as an active processor of information, whose behaviour is influenced by a rationally based decision – at least rational to them, even if it does not seem so to staff (Donovan and Blake, 1992). It is therefore important to explore patients' attitudes toward treatment: if we can anticipate and deal with any fears and doubts they have, we can better work with them to help them follow through on treatment. Good communication is aided by staff finding out what the patient's concerns and expectations are, rather than just gathering objective medical information. If expectations cannot be met, we need to explain why.

People often have misunderstandings about illness and treatment which can lead to apparent non-compliance. Ley (1979) found that patients often do not understand the information given by doctors, or fail to understand its significance. They also forget a substantial amount of information given. Ley's findings can be usefully translated into clinical practice. For example, important information should be presented early in a consultation, since the first third of an interview is remembered best. Also we should not present too much information in one session, since the proportion forgotten increases with the number of statements made. Other suggestions from Ley's research include categorizing information, using specific rather than general advice and avoiding medical jargon and technical terms.

Ross (1987) reported that first attenders at an STI clinic had a higher likelihood of non-compliance with treatment, apparently because they were less likely to see sexually transmitted disease as an illness than were those with previous infections. Redfern and Hutchinson (1994) found that women with repeated STIs had very different explanatory models for this than did health care professionals. The women did not necessarily attribute their condition to sexual behaviour at all. Staff and patients need to work towards a shared and accurate explanation for STIs in order to improve the likelihood of successful treatment and prevention.

Even with adequate information, emotional factors may affect compliance. Among women with abnormal cervical smears, Funke and Nicholson (1993) found that a moderate degree of anxiety about the smear test aided compliance with medical recommendations, whereas women who reported that they had not been able to cope with the abnormal result – who presumably had very high anxiety – were much less likely to comply with the advice given. Non-compliance has particular implications in GUM since if people do not complete a course of antibiotics, not only may the illness recur (often in a more resistant form) but it may be re-transmitted back and forth between partners.

Treatment may also be hindered by phobic anxiety about aspects of medical care. For example, fear of needles and syringes, or of specula, can prevent people from receiving adequate medical assessment and treatment. They can be helped by systematic desensitization programmes, which can often be implemented by nursing staff in consultation with a clinical psychologist.

Other psychological problems

Surveys suggest a high prevalence of general psychological difficulties among GUM clinic attenders. Catalan and colleagues (1981) found that 20% of a GUM clinic population could be categorized as 'psychiatric cases' as measured by the General Health Questionnaire (GHQ). This is comparable to rates found in other hospital outpatient populations. In a study of alcohol misuse in this population, Catalan, Day and Gallwey (1988) suggest that whether the prevalence is higher than in the general population is less important than that people happen to have come into contact with a medical facility where their problem could be recognized and appropriate advice offered. Fitzpatrick and colleagues (1987) found that 38% of GUM patients scored highly on the GHQ, indicating possible psychological disturbance, but that only 20% of such cases were also rated by the doctor as having psychological difficulties. These authors discuss variables that may limit or facilitate the communication of psychological distress. However, in another study Fitzpatrick, Frost and Ikkos (1986) found a significant association between high GHQ scores and patients' reports of concerns and worries about illness in relation to their presenting complaint. This suggests that much of the psychological disturbance found by this and other surveys of GUM clinics may represent temporary distress in relation to the presenting problem, and in most cases this is not necessarily abnormal or unwarranted. It may therefore be less likely to be noted by staff, being an understandable response to diagnosis. The level of distress found in GUM patients does not mean they necessarily need psychological help but it does imply that health care staff need to be sensitive to how patients are feeling, and not just focus on their medical problems.

However, as implied above by Catalan and colleagues, the fact that people have accessed a GUM service may provide an avenue into psychological therapy for those who need it. This may be particularly so for gay men and lesbians (or for those experiencing confusion/ambivalence about sexuality and sexual orientation), who may previously have found mainstream services unacceptably homophobic. As George (1993) points out, it is only a few decades since the dominant paradigms in clinical psychology and psychiatry defined homosexuality as pathological, and this may hinder gay men and lesbians from approaching conventional helping agencies for psychological support. Many people who access counselling services through GUM clinics are seeking help with psycho-social problems where the issue of HIV or STIs may not be of primary importance. People who are reluctant to present to their GPs with concerns about their sexuality may find GUM staff more approachable in this respect.

ROLE OF CLINICAL PSYCHOLOGY AND OTHER COUNSELLORS

As mentioned above in relation to HIV, not all patients with psychological difficulties will necessarily want or need to be referred for specialist counselling or psychotherapy. Indeed, an element of basic counselling can be seen as part of the job of all clinical staff, and doctors and nurses in GUM need good basic listening and communication skills. They should know how to present medical information – often including bad news – in a sympathetic and comprehensible way, and need to be alert to patients' concerns, whether directly or indirectly expressed. Nurses generally see every patient attending the clinic, and may be seen as more approachable and informal than medical staff. They therefore play a key role in putting patients at ease, identifying their psychological needs and helping them to access more specialist counselling staff where appropriate. Matocha and Waterhouse (1993) argue that:

Nursing practice addressing sexuality is a recognized part of providing holistic client care and may include assessing sexual health, providing anticipatory guidance about sexual development, validating normalcy, educating about sexuality and disease prevention, secondary prevention of disease of the reproductive organs, counselling clients who must adapt to changes in their usual forms of sexual expression, providing intensive therapy for sexual problems, and referring clients to other health care providers.

They cite Annon's (1974) model as providing a framework of four levels of intervention at which nurses may operate in sexuality counselling. This model enables nurses to assess the level of intervention they can offer and whether any further training is necessary. The first level is *permission*, and all nurses should be able to function at this level. It involves conveying to the patient that sexuality is a suitable subject for discussion, and giving assurance that their concerns or practices are normal. Most nurses can also intervene at the second *limited information* level, by giving factual information relevant to the patient's problems, and addressing general sexual concerns, questions, myths and misconceptions. Some nurses may have the additional training and experience to provide help at the third level of *specific suggestions* about sexual concerns and dysfunctions, but many patients requiring input at this level, and at the fourth level of *intensive therapy*, will need to be referred to an appropriate professional, e.g. a clinical psychologist or psychosexual counsellor. This is indicated when the nature or degree of someone's distress is greater than the doctor or nurse has the time or skills to deal with, and more intensive and longer-term support is needed. Ideally the psychologist or counsellor is an integral member of the multidisciplinary team and sees patients on-site, perhaps when they are attending for a medical appointment.

IMPACT OF THE WORK ON HEALTH CARE STAFF

The stigma of GUM is not a problem for patients only. It can place an additional strain on health care staff working in this area. Coleman and Etchegoyen (1992) point out aspects of the STI clinic which can affect the presentation of problems. For example, the isolation of the clinic and the level of confidentiality can lead to an atmosphere of secrecy which may cause people to deny their feelings or the seriousness of their problems. It can also lead to staff being less connected with their professional network of colleagues.

HIV work in particular is likely to affect staff personally in various ways; this needs to be acknowledged and dealt with in order for the staff to be fully effective as helpers. Working with people with life-threatening illness, including experiencing deaths among our patients, is distressing in itself. It also brings us face to face with the fact of our own mortality and may raise questions and concerns about our own risk of HIV infection. There can be two reactions to this. We may become overinvolved, and find that the patient's problems stimulate so much personal distress that we can no longer be objective, and find the work overwhelming. At the other extreme, we may overdistance ourselves, in order to deny the threat to us, and this prevents us from fully engaging when talking to patients about their needs and concerns. In a survey of various health care staff, Barbour (1995) found that HIV was not necessarily a more stressful speciality in itself; however, many staff reported criticism and hostility from family, friends, and colleagues in other fields, especially if they had specifically chosen to work in this speciality.

CONCLUSION

Genitourinary medicine cannot be fully effective without due attention to the psychological needs of patients. This is important both in order to provide holistic care and also to facilitate people coming back for necessary treatment and 'test of cure' if applicable. Some of the psychological issues involved are the same as those of any medical setting, and others are specific to particular aspects of this setting, where very private and socially taboo issues need to be addressed. Our concern for confidentiality and anonymity must not lead us to respond impersonally to the people who come to us for care. The issues discussed above should therefore be borne in mind when reading the more clinically oriented chapters in this book.

REFERENCES

Annon, J.S. (1974) *The Behavioral Treatment of Sexual Problems*, Enabling Systems, Honolulu.

Arnold, R.P., Rogers, D. and Cook, D.A.G. (1990) Medical problems of adults who were sexually abused in childhood. *British Medical Journal, 17 March* **300** pp. 705–8.

Barbour, R. (1995) The implications of HIV/AIDS for a range of workers in the Scottish context. *AIDS CARE*, **7**(4), 521–35.

Bassuk, E. (1980) A crisis theory perspective on rape, in *The Rape Crisis Intervention Handbook* (ed. S.L. McCombie), Plenum Press, New York, pp. 121–9.

Beaman, M.L. and Strader, M.K. (1989) STD patients' knowledge about AIDS and attitudes toward condom use. *Journal of Community Health Nursing*, **6**(5), 155–64.

Bell, S., Porter, M., Kitchener, H. *et al.* (1995) Psychological response to cervical screening. *Preventive Medicine*, **24**(6), 610–16.

Bennetts, A., Irwig, L., Oldenburg, B. *et al.* (1995) PEAPS-Q: a questionnaire to measure the psychosocial effects of having an abnormal pap smear. Psychosocial Effects of Abnormal Pap Smears Questionnaire. *Journal of Clinical Epidemiology*, **48**(10), 1235–43.

Bor, R. and Miller, R. (1988) Addressing 'dreaded issues': a description of a unique counselling intervention with patients with AIDS/HIV. *Counselling Psychology Quarterly*, **1**, 397–406.

Burgess, A.W. and Holmstrom, L.L. (1974) Rape trauma syndrome. *American Journal of Psychiatry*, **31**(9), 981–6.

Cahill, C., Llewelyn, S.P. and Pearson, C. (1991) Long-term effects of sexual abuse which occurred in childhood: a review. *British Journal of Clinical Psychology*, **30**, 117–30.

Carney, O., Ross, E., Ikkos, G. and Mindel, A. (1993) The effect of suppressive oral acyclovir on the psychological morbidity associated with recurrent genital herpes. *Genitourinary Medicine*, **69**(6), 457–9.

Catalan, J., Bradley, M., Gallwey, J. and Hawton, K. (1981) Sexual dysfunction and psychiatric morbidity in patients attending a clinic for sexually transmitted diseases. *British Journal of Psychiatry*, **138**, 292–6.

Catalan, J., Day, A. and Gallwey, J. (1988) Alcohol misuse in patients attending a genitourinary clinic. *Alcohol and Alcoholism*, **23**(5), 421–8.

Chandler, M.G. (1996) Genital warts: a study of patient anxiety and information needs. *British Journal of Nursing*, **5**(3), 174–9.

Coleman, R. and Etchegoyen, A. (1992) The psychodynamics of the STD clinic: secrecy, splitting and isolation. *British Journal of Medical Psychology*, **65**(4), 319–26.

Dalkvist, J., Wahlin, T.B., Bartsch, E. and Forsbeck, M. (1995) Herpes simplex and mood: a prospective study. *Psychosomatic Medicine*, **57**(2), 127–37.

Donovan, J.L. and Blake, D.R. (1992) Patient non-compliance: deviance or reasoned decision-making? *Social Science and Medicine*, **34**(5), 507–13.

Drob, S., Loemer, M. and Lifshutz, H. (1985) Genital herpes: the psychological consequences. *British Journal of Medical Psychology*, **58**, 307–15.

Evans, D. and Farquhar, C. (1996) An interview based approach to seeking user views in genitourinary medicine. *Genitourinary Medicine*, **72**(3), 223–6.

Faxelid, E. and Krantz, I. (1993) Experiences of disease and treatment among chlamydia patients. *Scandinavian Journal of Caring Sciences*, **7**(3), 169–73.

Filiberti, A., Tamburini, M., Stefanon, B. *et al.* (1993) Psychological aspects of genital human papillomavirus infection: a preliminary report. *Journal of Psychosomatic Obstetrics and Gynaecology*, **14**(2), 145–52.

Fishbein, M. and Ajzen, I. (1975) *Belief, Attitude, Intention and Behaviour: An Introduction to Theory and Research*, Addison-Wesley, Reading, MA.

Fitzpatrick, R., Frost, D. and Ikkos, G. (1986) Survey of psychological disturbance in patients attending a sexually transmitted disease clinic. *Genitourinary Medicine*, **62**, 111–15.

Fitzpatrick, R., Ikkos, G., Frost, D. and Nazeer, S. (1987) The assessment of patients' distress in genito-urinary medicine clinics. *Social Science and Medicine*, **25**(11), 1197–203.

Funke, B.L. and Nicholson, M.E. (1993) Factors affecting patient compliance among women with abnormal Pap smears. *Patient Education and Counseling*, **20**(1), 5–15.

George, H. (1993) Sex, love and relationships: issues and problems for gay men in the AIDS era, in *Psychological Perspectives on Sexual Problems* (eds J.M. Ussher and C.D. Baker), Routledge, London.

Glaser, J.B., Hammerschlag, M.R. and McCormack, W.M. (1989) Epidemiology of sexually transmitted diseases in rape victims. *Review of Infectious Diseases*, **11**(2), 246–54.

Gordon, P. (1987) Psychosexual counselling in an STD clinic. *British Journal of Sexual Medicine*, July, 199–203.

Green, J. and McCreaner, A. (eds) (1996) *Counselling in HIV infection and AIDS*, 2nd edn, Blackwell Science, Oxford.

Helsen, K. and Kinghorn, G.R. (1991) Extragenital complication of genital herpes. *British Journal of Sexual Medicine*, Spring, 8–11.

Hillman, R.J., Tomlinson, D., McMillan, A. *et al.* (1990) Sexual assault of men: a series. *Genitourinary Medicine*, **66**, 247–50.

Kocsis, A. (1996) AIDS dementia – counselling issues, in Green and McCreaner (1996), op. cit.

Koss, M.P. (1993) Rape – scope, impact, interventions, and public policy responses. *American Psychologist*, **48**(10), 1061–9.

Ley, P. (1979) Memory for medical information. *British Journal of Social and Clinical Psychology*, **18**, 245–55.

Marteau, T.M., Kidd, J., Cuddeford, L. and Walker, P. (1996) Reducing anxiety in women referred for colposcopy using an information booklet. *British Journal of Health Psychology*, **1**(2), 181–9.

Matocha, L.K. and Waterhouse, J.K. (1993) Current nursing practice related to sexuality. *Research in Nursing and Health*, **16**, 371–8.

Miller, D., Acton, T.M.G. and Hedge, B. (1988) Th worried well: their identification and management. *Journal of the Royal College of Physicians of London*, **22**(3), 158–64.

Munday, P.E. (1990) Genitourinary medicine services: consumers' views. *Genitourinary Medicine*, **66**, 108–11.

Redfern, N. and Hutchinson, S. (1994) Women's experiences of repetitively contracting sexually transmitted diseases. *Health Care for Women International*, **15**(5), 423–33.

Roffman, R.A., Gordon, J.R. and Craver, J.N. (1987) AIDS risk reduction: preventing relapse to unsafe sex. Paper presented at World Congress of Behaviour Therapy, Edinburgh.

Ross, M.W. (1987) Illness behaviour among patients attending a sexually transmitted disease clinic. *Sexually Transmitted Diseases*, **14**(3), 174–9.

Stronks, D.L., Rijpma, S.E., Passchier, J. *et al.* (1993) Psychological consequences of genital herpes, an exploratory study with a gonorrhea control-group. *Psychological Reports*, **73**(2), 395–400.

Swanson, J.M., Dibble, S.L. and Chenitz, W.C. (1995) Clinical features and psychosocial factors in young adults with genital herpes. *Image – The Journal of Nursing Scholarship*, **27**(1), 16–22.

Tomaino-Brunner, C., Freda, M.C. and Runowicz, C.D. (1996) 'I hope I don't have cancer': colposcopy and minority women. *Oncology Nursing Forum*, **23**(1), 39–44.

Voog, E. and Lowhagen, G.B. (1992) Follow-up of men with genital papilloma virus infection. Psychosocial aspects. *Acta Dermato-Venereologica*, **72**(3), 185–6.

Zverina, J., Lachman, M., Pondelickova, J. and Vanek, J. (1987) The occurrence of atypical sexual experience among various female patient groups. *Archives of Sexual Behaviour*, **16**(4), 321–6.

5 The male and female reproductive systems

Dinah Gould

OBJECTIVES

1. To name the male and female reproductive structures.
2. To state which types of tissue within the male and female reproductive systems are particularly susceptible to infection.
3. To state where the tissues are located.
4. To explain the general effects of infection on the male and female arising as a consequence of sexually transmitted infection.

SUMMARY

The purpose of this chapter is to outline the structure and function of the healthy male and female reproductive organs, pointing out the tissues particularly susceptible to infection. The damage caused by infection is indicated and the ways in which infection is excluded in the healthy individual are explained.

INTRODUCTION

The design of the human body directly affects its ability to function. Thus knowledge of the normal structure and function of the male and female reproductive organs is essential before it is possible to appreciate the changes that accompany acute and chronic infections caused by sexually transmitted agents.

THE MALE REPRODUCTIVE SYSTEM

The organs of the male reproductive system are designed to permit the following functions:

- sexual arousal;
- the production of male gametes (spermatozoa) and their transfer to the female during sexual intercourse;
- the production of the male sex hormones (androgens).

The male reproductive tract consists of the urethra, penis and scrotum and the following paired structures (see Figure 5.1).

- testes (male gonads)
- epididymis
- vasa deferentia
- ejaculatory ducts
- prostate gland
- bulbo-urethral glands

The testes

The testes are the male gonads responsible for secreting the male hormones, principally testosterone, and for producing sperm. Each is approximately 4.5 cm long and 2.5 cm in diameter. The testes arise in the abdomen during embryonic development and descend into the scrotum via the inguinal canals during the eighth month of pregnancy.

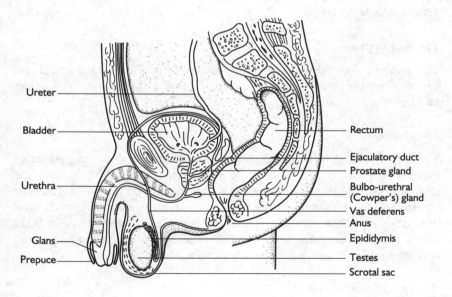

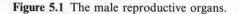

Figure 5.1 The male reproductive organs.

The spermatic cord, consisting of the spermatic artery, the spermatic vein and nerve descend with each testicle.

Occasionally the testicles fail to descend into the scrotum, a situation that must be corrected surgically to avoid the risk of malignant change which sometimes occurs in the undescended testicle. A second reason is to avoid sterility: sperm production requires a temperature 2–3°C cooler than body temperature. Muscular contraction occurs to alter the position of the scrotum in response to temperature changes. For example, heat causes the scrotum to hang loosely away from the body while cold stimulates muscular contraction, moving the scrotum closer to the body.

Each testicle occupies a separate compartment within the scrotum. Additionally each testicle is covered by two layers of tissue:

- the tunica vaginalis—a double serous layer;
- the tunica albuginea, which forms the septae dividing each testicle into 200–300 lobules.

The lobules

Each lobule is a wedge-shaped structure. Individual lobules contain the highly convoluted seminiferous tubules. These are the sites of sperm production (spermatogenesis). The interstitial (Leydig) cells also found within the seminiferous tubules secrete the androgens. The principal androgen is testosterone.

The duct system

The seminiferous tubules from the lobules form the tubuli recti. These converge on the rete testis, which in turn unite with the efferent ductules and the epididymis.

The epididymis

The epididymis is a convoluted tube 6 m long coiled on the posterior surface of each testicle. Sperm are carried to the epididymis from the seminiferous tubules via the rete testis and the efferent ductules. They are transferred by muscular contractions because they are still immature at this stage and lack motility. Their journey along the epididymis takes about three weeks. During this time the sperm reach maturity and become motile.

The vas deferens

The vas deferens continues from the epididymis. It is a tube approximately 45 cm long, travelling in the spermatic cord to enter the pelvic cavity. Each of the vasa deferentia runs in front of the pubic bone, over the ureter and behind the bladder. Here they dilate to form the ampulla. At ejaculation a layer of muscle in the wall of the vas deferens contracts rapidly. This conveys mature spermatozoa into the urethra.

The seminal vesicles

The seminal vesicles are tubular glands with muscular walls lined with secretory epithelium. The function of their secretion, a viscous, alkaline fluid, is to help nourish the spermatozoa. Secretion enters the ampullae of the vasa deferentia via the two ejaculatory ducts as they pass through the prostate gland. Approximately 60% of the volume of the semen consists of secretion from the seminal vesicles.

The prostate gland

The prostate gland surrounds the first part of the male urethra. It consists of numerous segments of glandular tissue, fibrous and muscular tissue, all enclosed within a capsule. Secretion from the prostate gland is added to the semen during ejaculation. It is a thin, watery solution, thought to enhance the motility of the spermatozoa and to increase the acidic pH of the vagina, which is hostile to sperm. Prostatic enlargement (hypertrophy) is common from mid-life onwards. Males in this age group frequently experience difficulty passing urine, with retention developing in severe cases. Benign hypertrophy is most likely to be apparent in men of sixty or older, but malignant tumours of the prostate may develop in younger men. Prostatic cancer is one of the most common causes of male mortality from malignancy in the UK, so any complaints made by patients must be investigated thoroughly.

The penis

The penis consists of three columns of erectile tissue. These contain vascular spaces, connective tissue and involuntary muscle and a rich supply of blood vessels and autonomic nerves. During sexual excitement the vascular spaces become filled with blood, resulting in erection. Impaired circulation or damage to the nervous supply may result in physiological impotence.

A fold of skin called the prepuce (foreskin) surrounds the tip of the penis. The prepuce attaches to the neck of the penis, continuing over the glans (head) of the penis which surrounds the external urethral meatus. A number of tiny glands open on to the surface of the glans penis. Their secretion is a waxy material called smegma, which provides an ideal medium for bacterial growth. Mild infections caused by a variety of microorganisms are therefore common at this site, especially in males who have not been circumcised. Balanitis (infection of the head of the penis) is particularly common in patients with diabetes mellitus. The urine should be tested for the presence of glucose in individuals who report recurrent balanitis.

The urethra

The male urethra extends from the urinary bladder to the tip of the penis. It is long compared to the female urethra (15–20 cm). Thus infections of the urinary tract are less common in males than females, as invading organisms have further to travel before reaching the bladder. The male urethra can be divided into three anatomical regions:

- The prostatic urethra, which passes through the prostate gland.
- The membranous urethra—the short segment penetrating the muscular floor of the pelvic cavity. It is the narrowest part of the male urethra and, because it is relatively inelastic, may tear during injuries to the perineum.
- The penile urethra extends from the border of the pelvic floor, along the entire length of the penis to the external urethral meatus.

The bulbo-urethral glands

The bulbo-urethral (Cowper's) glands are tiny paired glands situated below the prostate gland. They empty their secretions into the bulb of the urethra. Their function is lubrication: they secrete small quantities of lubricating fluid into the urethra before ejaculation.

Infections in the male reproductive tract

In men the urethra, its glands, the prostate glands, the seminal vesicle and the epididymes are at particular risk of damage from sexually transmitted agents, especially *Neisseria gonorrhoeae*, because they are lined with delicate columnar epithelium which is readily invaded by pathogens (See Chapter 8). Ascending infection is unlikely to affect the bladder in males or females because of its tougher epithelial lining (pseudostratified epithelium). If untreated, infection in the male can cause urethral stricture and dysuria and may ascend to involve the seminiferous tubules, eventually resulting in infertility.

THE FEMALE REPRODUCTIVE SYSTEM

The organs of the female reproductive system are designed to permit the following functions:

- production of the female sex steroids (oestrogen and progesterone)
- sexual arousal by lubrication of the female genitalia
- coitus
- production of female gametes (ova)
- safe development of the embryo and fetus
- parturition

All these functions depend on the exclusion of infection from the female reproductive tract.

The external female genitalia [vulva]

The vulva consists of the following structures (see Figure 5.2):

- the mons pubis, a pad of fatty tissue situated over the symphysis pubis and covered with pubic hair;
- the labia majora; skin-covered areas containing numerous sebaceous glands (pubic hair covers their outer but not their inner aspect);
- the labia minora, two smaller, skin-covered folds protected by the labia majora;
- the clitoris; the female analogue of the penis and the seat of sexual arousal, containing erectile tissue and a rich nervous supply.

The vestibule

This is the area within the labia minora. As well as the clitoris, the vestibule contains the openings of the urethra and the vagina.

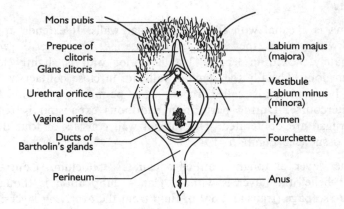

Figure 5.2 The vulva.

The greater vestibular (Bartholin's) glands

The function of these paired glands is to lubricate the vestibule during sexual arousal. They lie just behind the vestibule, covered with skin and muscle, with a duct carrying secretion from each to the exterior. Bartholin's glands cannot usually be palpated, but occasionally a duct may become blocked, giving rise to a swelling which can be felt beneath the skin. Structurally, Bartholin's glands are very similar to the bulbo-urethral glands in the male and are susceptible to infection, especially if a duct has become blocked. The result is a painful abscess which must be opened surgically to facilitate drainage (marsupialization). Bartholinitis may be caused by many different bacteria including *Neisseria gonorrhoeae*.

The lesser vestibular (Skene's) glands

These small paired glands open on to the urethral meatus, providing lubrication. Again, they are susceptible to infection.

The internal female genitalia

The internal organs of the female reproductive tract (Figure 5.3) consist of:

- vagina
- uterus
- uterine (Fallopian) tubes
- ovaries

The vagina

The vagina is a canal with fibrous, muscular walls. It extends upwards and backwards from the vulva to the uterus. The anterior wall is approximately 7.5 cm in length. The posterior wall is slightly longer, about 9 cm long. Usually the vaginal walls are in close contact with one another, lying in folds called rugae. This permits expansion during sexual intercourse. During parturition enormous expansion is required and the rugae are obliterated. The vaginal wall consists of four distinct layers of tissue (see Figure 5.4):

- An inner layer of tough stratified squamous epithelium. Contrary to popular belief this layer is without glands: lubrication is thought to occur by seepage (transudation) of fluid from the overlying layers.
- A layer of white, spongy areolar connective tissue. This contains the vascular and nervous supply.

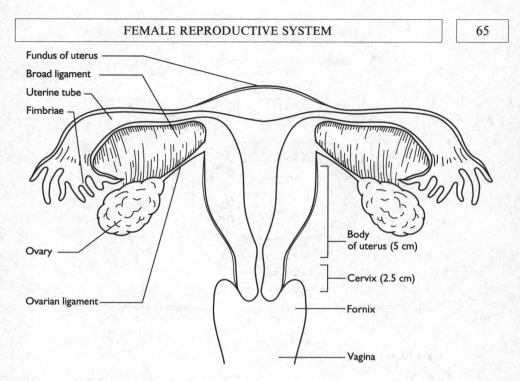

Fundus of uterus

Broad ligament

Uterine tube

Fimbriae

Ovary

Ovarian ligament

Body of uterus (5 cm)

Cervix (2.5 cm)

Fornix

Vagina

Figure 5.3 The internal female reproductive system.

- A layer of smooth (involuntary) muscle.
- An outer coat of tough, fibrous connective tissue to protect the inner structures. This blends with the pelvic fascia.

The cervix dips down into the top of the vagina, to form a gutter called the fornices. The posterior fornix is deeper than the anterior fornix. This is because of the sloping position of the vaginal vault. During intercourse, semen is deposited chiefly into the posterior fornix. Sperm may survive here for between three and five days, protected by the alkaline mucus secreted by glands in the cervical epithelium. Recent research indicates that conception is most likely if intercourse occurs in the days immediately before ovulation (days 11–14) of a 28 day menstrual cycle (Wilcox, Weinberg and Baird, 1995). Figure 5.5 shows the close anatomical relationship between the vagina, the bladder and the rectum. This is of clinical significance, as spread of neoplastic cells from the cervix can occur locally, affecting other structures.

Throughout the reproductive years the vagina is protected against infection by secretions from the cervix. The cells of the stratified squamous epithelium lining the vagina are tough and resist invasion by microorganisms. In addition, these cells are continually shed and release glycogen, a

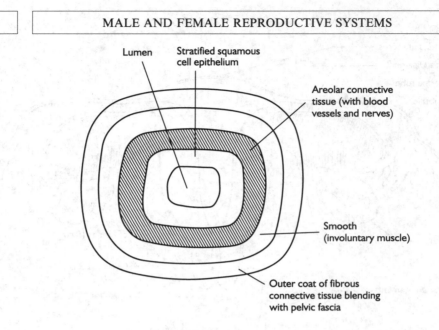

Lumen

Stratified squamous cell epithelium

Areolar connective tissue (with blood vessels and nerves)

Smooth (involuntary muscle)

Outer coat of fibrous connective tissue blending with pelvic fascia

Figure 5.4 The vaginal wall.

complex carbohydrate which is metabolized by a resident population of vaginal bacteria belonging to the lactobacillus group. The lactobacilli convert glycogen to lactic acid, so the vaginal environment is maintained at a relatively low pH (pH 4–5), inhibiting the growth of foreign micro-organisms. The growth and intense metabolic activity of the vaginal epithe-lium are maintained by oestrogen. Before the menarche, in the absence of oestrogen, the vaginal epithelium is thinner and more prone to infection. After the menopause, oestrogen levels decline and the vaginal epithelium atrophies: overgrowth by invading microorganisms is commonplace, leading to atrophic vaginitis. This can be successfully treated by the topical application of oestrogen cream in women for whom hormone replacement therapy (HRT) is contra-indicated and for those who do not wish to receive it. Pregnancy sometimes alters vaginal pH, disturbing the normal vaginal flora. Infection may supervene. Candida infection is common during preg-nancy and has been associated with metabolic disorders, notably diabetes mellitus. It may also develop as a result of treatment with antibiotics because they destroy the normal vaginal bacteria. (See Chapter 13.)

Although the vaginal wall successfully excludes most pathogens, minute abrasions may allow access to toxins produced by *Staphylococcus aureus*. These bacteria are carried as part of the normal skin flora by approxi-mately 30% of the healthy population (Gould and Chamberlain, 1995).

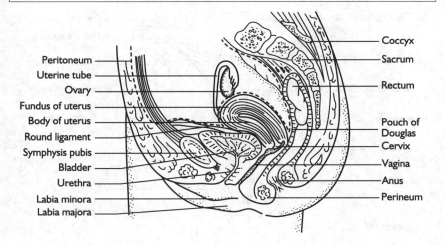

Figure 5.5 Sagittal section of the female reproductive system.

The usual sites of carriage include the axillae, throat, nares and the perineum. Spread is by the contact route, especially via hands (Gould and Chamberlain, 1995). Transfer to the vaginal epithelium probably occurs when a tampon is changed. As the tampon absorbs the menstrual flow, ideal conditions are created for bacterial multiplication. The toxins gain access to the bloodstream via minute ulcerations in the epithelium caused by the tampon, especially if superabsorbent varieties are used, because of their drying effect. In the bloodstream the toxins give rise to a severe generalised illness characterized by: pyrexia, rash, vomiting, headache, diarrhoea and sore throat. In the most severe cases dehydration and hypotension rapidly lead to shock. Toxic shock syndrome is an uncommon condition, but has received widespread coverage by the media because occasional fatalities have occurred. Women who are concerned can be given the following advice:

- Wash hands carefully before as well as after inserting a tampon.
- Use a tampon of the correct absorbency: risks accrue when a more absorbent variety or larger size than necessary is employed.
- Change the tampon frequently (4–6 hours).
- Take care not to forget about tampons when menstruation ceases.

The uterus

The uterus is a hollow, muscular organ, uniquely designed to shelter the embryo and fetus throughout pregnancy and to expel the infant by means

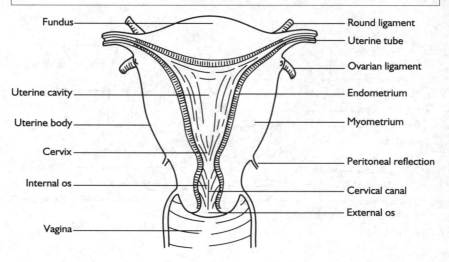

Figure 5.6 The uterus.

of powerful muscular contractions during parturition. Anatomically it is divided into a cervix (neck), which projects down into the vagina, and a corpus (body). In the healthy, non-pregnant state the entire uterus is typically 7.5 cm long and 5.5 cm wide. The walls are approximately 1.2 cm in thickness and almost obliterate the uterine cavity (see Figure 5.6).

The cervix

Before puberty the cervical canal and the surface of the cervix projecting into the vagina are both covered with a layer of columnar epithelial cells. This type of tissue is extremely delicate and may succumb to infection. At puberty the columnar epithelial cells lining the cervical os (opening) become replaced with tougher squamous epithelial cells and the risk of infection and trauma is reduced. Columnar cells still line the cervical canal, producing mucus secretions. However, in some women the squamous layer may become overgrown with the delicate columnar cells. This condition, known as cervical erosion, is benign but places the woman at greater risk of developing infection. Invading microorganisms unable to gain a foothold in the tough squamous epithelium of the vagina frequently establish themselves in the columnar cells of the cervix; typical examples of infections behaving in this manner are gonorrhoea and chlamydial infections (see Chapters 7 and 8). Women taking the contraceptive pill seem to be particularly at risk of developing cervical erosion.

The corpus

The body of the uterus consists of a thick muscular wall (myometrium) lined with endometrium. Endometrium is an epithelial tissue containing numerous glands.

The endometrium

The endometrium consists of two layers: a permanent basal layer (stratum basalis) and an upper layer (stratum functionalis) shed during menstruation, approximately every 28 days throughout the reproductive years. The endometrial changes occurring during the menstrual cycle are as follows:

- *Menstruation.* Beginning on day 1 of the cycle, over a period of about five days the superficial endometrial layer is shed, leaving the basal layer.
- *The proliferative phase.* From about day 5 of the cycle a few cells from the old superficial layer sheltered deep within the endometrial glands of the basal layer begin to multiply, leading to progressive thickening and increased vasculation as ovulation approaches. Ovulation occurs at the midpoint of the typical 28 day cycle, 14 days before the commencement of menstruation in *any* cycle, irrespective of its length.
- *The secretory phase.* Following ovulation, oestrogen continues to promote endometrial development. The release of progesterone from the corpus luteum (cells that surrounded the ovum in the ovary) prepares the endometrium to receive a fertilized egg. The endometrial blood supply further increases and the endometrial glands, now highly coiled, secrete glycogen to provide nourishment. If implantation does not occur, the corpus luteum degenerates, the supply of hormones ceases abruptly and menstruation follows.

Note the rapidity with which the stratum basalis becomes re-epithelialized following menstruation. Thus the threat of infection into the exposed tissue is minimized. In contrast, the separation of the placenta at parturition exposes a large raw area which is at risk from invading microorganisms. The risk of puerperal infection must be reduced by keeping invasive interventions (e.g. vaginal examination) to a minimum before delivery and by paying strict attention to asepsis before and after the baby is born.

The menstrual cycle is controlled by a series of complex interactions between hormones secreted from the anterior pituitary gland and the ovaries. Detailed descriptions lie beyond the scope of this specialized book, but may be found in general anatomy and physiology texts (Hubbard and Mechan, 1997). A knowledge of the changes that occur throughout the normal menstrual cycle and the ability to recognize and assess abnormal signs and symptoms are both important for the nurse working in the GU clinic. Menorrhagia, the excessive, regular loss of menstrual blood—one of the most common reasons for referral to a gynaecologist—is frequently painful as well as inconvenient and if severe may lead to anaemia (Coulter, McPherson and Vessey, 1988). Women who have been anxious about symptoms for some time may take this opportunity to mention them, or the occurrence of abnormalities may become evident during clinic attendance. Appropriate referral will then be possible.

The uterine (Fallopian) tubes

The two uterine (Fallopian) tubes project laterally from the fundus (upper part) of the uterus, extending from their points of insertion (the cornuae) towards the pelvic walls. Each is approximately 10 cm long with an extremely narrow diameter. The uterine tubes terminate in a series of fine fimbriae which open in close proximity to the ovarian surfaces, although there is no direct contact between the two organs. They are delicate, highly specialised structures, designed to convey the sperm towards the ovary while nourishing the ova during their passage towards the uterus (see Figure 5.7). Their epithelial lining consists of delicate ciliated columnar cells interspersed with secretory cells. The rhythmic beating of the cilia and peristaltic contractions in the muscular walls of the uterine tubes propel the ova towards the uterus while the secretory cells provide nourishment. In health, fertilization usually occurs in the slightly expanded part of the tube called the ampulla. By the time the conceptus reaches the endometrium it has undergone a number of cellular divisions into a multicellular morula.

Despite their anatomical position deep within the pelvic cavity, the uterine tubes are at high risk of infection because of the fine structure of their epithelial lining. Infection may ascend from the vagina and cervix or, more rarely, it may enter from the pelvic cavity via the open fimbriated ends of the tubes. The organisms responsible for gonorrhoea and non-specific urethritis frequently migrate from the cervix to the uterine tubes, while bacteria causing peritonitis may invade via the fimbriae. (See Chapter 10.)

Salpingitis

Salpingitis is an extremely damaging infection which can profoundly affect fertility and general health (see also Chapter 10). Infection gives rise to inflammation and the formation of scar tissue. In acute cases purulent material accumulates to form an abscess (pyosalpinx). As a result the victim will experience acute pelvic pain, pyrexia and malaise. Chronic infections give rise to lower-grade pyrexia, poorly localized

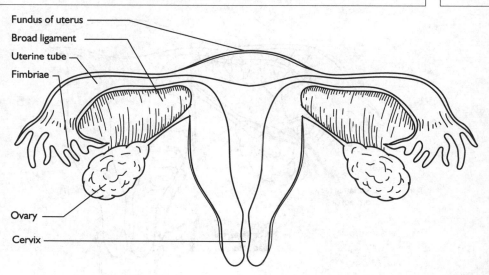

Fundus of uterus
Broad ligament
Uterine tube
Fimbriae
Ovary
Cervix

Figure 5.7 The uterine (Fallopian) tubes.

pelvic pain and general, sometimes vague complaints of feeling unwell. In both cases, scarring will lead to occlusion of the fimbriae and interfere with the normal movements of the uterine tubes, which increase at the time of ovulation and when the ovum is moving towards the uterus. Fertility is impaired. Adhesions may prevent encounter between the ovum and sperm, or the ovum, if fertilized, may implant at an extrauterine site, most commonly the ampulla, resulting in an ectopic pregnancy. At any point in time 9–14% of women of childbearing age seek medical help because they are experiencing difficulty becoming pregnant (Templeton, Fraser and Thompson, 1990) and of these approximately 14% have tubal damage (Hull, Glazner and Kelly, 1985). Diagnosis and treatment have been reported as stressful and are not straightforward: the most effective forms of treatment for subfertility caused by tubal damage are assisted conception techniques such as *in vitro* fertilization (Alder, 1985). These are available only at selected centres, success rates are variable and treatment is costly whether provided by the NHS or privately funded by the individual (Human Fertilisation Embryology Authority, 1992). In contrast, tubal repair operations frequently provide disappointing results unless damage is mild (Winston and Margara, 1991). The rate of ectopic pregnancy is approximately 0.8% in the general population in the UK, this event sometimes occurring after attempts to repair tubal damage. It is a major cause of maternal

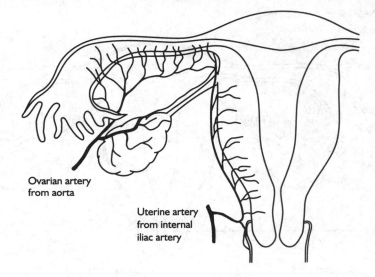

Ovarian artery
from aorta

Uterine artery
from internal
iliac artery

Figure 5.8 Blood supply to the female pelvic organs.

morbidity and mortality (Lavy, Diamond and DeCherney, 1987). This is because erosion of the tubal wall by the trophoblast may lead to considerable bleeding; the uterine tubes being well vasculated (see Figure 5.8).

The ovaries

The ovaries (female gonads) lie deep within the pelvic cavity, with their surfaces positioned closely to the fimbriae of the uterine tubes. Their function is to produce ova and the female sex steroids oestrogen and progesterone. Each consists of an outer epithelial layer enclosing connective tissue containing the Graffian follicles which shelter the ova. Infection is uncommon, but may occasionally occur as a complication of pelvic inflammatory disease.

The female urethra

The female urethra is much shorter (4 cm) than that of the male so the urinary tract is less protected from infections, which are correspondingly more common. The tissue is under oestrogenic control, so withdrawal of oestrogen at the menopause may lead to atrophy and discomfort.

GLOSSARY

Bartholin's glands	Paired glands responsible for secreting a lubricating fluid during sexual arousal
Cervix	Narrow lower portion of the uterus projecting down into the vagina
Endometrium	Uterine lining
Epididymis	Long, convoluted tube carrying sperm from the testes to the vas deferens
Myometrium	Muscular wall of the uterus
Ovary	Female gonad which produces eggs and hormone (oestrogen and progesterone)
Pyosalpinx	Pus in the uterine (Fallopian) tube; an abscess
Salpingitis	Inflammation of the uterine tubes
Sterility	Absence of fertility
Subfertility	Impaired fertility
Testes	The male gonads which produce sperm and hormones (androgens)
Uterine (Fallopian) tube	Fine tube allowing the passage of the egg (ovum) from the ovary to the uterus
Vas deferens	Duct that carries sperm from the epididymis and the testes to the urethra

REFERENCES

Alder, T. (1985) Patient reaction to IVF treatment. *Lancet*, **i**, 168–9.

Coulter, A. McPherson, K. and Vessey M. (1988) Do British women undergo too many or too few hysterectomies? *Social Science and Medicine*, **27**, 987–94.

Gould, D. (1986) *Nursing Care of Women*, Prentice Hall, Hemel Hempstead.

Gould, D.J. and Chamberlain, A. (1995) *Staphylococcus aureus*: a review of the literature. *Journal of Clinical Nursing*, **4**, 5–12.

Hubbard, J. and Mechan, D. (1997) *The Physiology of Health and Illness*. Stanley Thornes (Publishers) Ltd.

Hull, M.G.R., Glazner, C.M. and Kelly, N.J. (1985) Population study of causes of treatment and outcomes of infertility. *British Medical Journal*, **291**, 1693–7.

Human Fertilisation Embryology Authority (1992) Annual Report.

Lavy, G., Diamond, M.P. and DeCherney, A.H. (1987) Ectopic pregnancy: its relationship to tubal reconstructive surgery. *Fertility and Sterility*, **47**, 543–4.

Templeton, A., Fraser, C. and Thompson, B. (1990) The epidemiology of infertility in Aberdeen. *British Medical Journal*, **301**, 148–52.

Wilcox, A.J., Weinberg, C.R. and Baird, D.D. (1995) Timing of sexual intercourse in relation to ovulation. *New England Journal of Medicine*, **333**, 1517–21.

Winston, R.M. and Margara, R.A. (1991) Microsurgical salpingostomy is not an obsolete procedure. *British Journal of Obstetrics and Gynaecology*, **98**, 637–42.

Genital ulceration

6

OBJECTIVES

1. To describe the microbiology of genital ulcer disease.
2. To recognize the signs and symptoms of syphilis and other ulcerative conditions.
3. To explain the route of transmission for the genital ulcerative infections.
4. To describe the consequences of untreated syphilis infection.
5. To identify the main techniques used to diagnose syphilis and the other genital ulcerative infections.
6. To list the common treatment regimes for all the genital ulcerative conditions.
7. To explain the importance of follow-up and contact tracing for these infections.

SUMMARY

An ulcer is a local loss of surface covering or epithelium and sometimes deeper tissue in the skin. The loss of the surface may lead to infection and further tissue damage. In the case of genital ulceration there is often an infective cause and once the ulcer appears a secondary infection may set in. Genital ulceration is significant in the transmission of other infections such as HIV due to breach of the skin as a natural defence against such organisms.

Genital ulceration has five main causes:

- syphilis
- *Herpes simplex*
- chancroid
- granuloma inguinale
- lymphogranuloma venereum

These will be considered in turn in this chapter. As syphilis and *Herpes simplex* are the most common of the ulcerative conditions observed in GUM clinics in this country these will be considered in most detail. *Herpes simplex* is fully described in Chapter 12.

SYPHILIS

Epidemiology

In the United Kingdom the incidence of syphilis has declined gradually and has remained steady for the past decade (Department of Health, 1995). In England there were only 304 cases of infective syphilis reported in 1994, 64% of these being men, 20% of those cases homosexually acquired. The epidemiology of syphilis since the beginning of the century is examined more closely in Chapter 3.

Microbiology

Spirochetes are free-living parasitic or pathogenic bacteria of an unusual shape. There are three main species of interest in GUM:

- *Treponema pallidum* causing syphilis
- *Treponema pertenue* causing yaws
- *Treponema carateum* causing pinta.

The latter two are tropical diseases, with different clinical manifestations to those of syphilis. Serology tests, however, appear similar in all three infections, highlighting the need for careful history taking.

Treponema pallidum has a corkscrew appearance of fine, regular spirals and is about 5–15 μm in length and 0.25 μm in width. They are motile and have an axial filament around which the bacteria twists, giving its characteristic shape. The incubation period is usually 2–4 weeks, the full range being 9–90 days.

Transmission

Syphilis is usually sexually transmitted but can also be transmitted by close contact with moist mucosal or cutaneous lesions. It can also be passed from mother to child during pregnancy as early as the ninth week of pregnancy and this may occur shortly after the mother has become infected herself (Chang, 1995). Untreated syphilis remains a potential source of infection to future pregnancies for up to eight years, resulting in congenital syphilis. The usual period of infectivity does not last beyond two years. After this the disease may remain active but bacteraemia does not occur.

Signs and symptoms

Primary stage

At the initial stage a small ulcer known as a 'chancre' may appear at the site of spirochete penetration. This is usually ovoid with a regular, clearly defined, punched-out margin. Granulation tissue appears at the centre and is usually painless unless secondary infection is present. If untreated, the ulcer will heal within a few weeks, sometimes leaving only a small scar. Common sites for the appearance of chancres are, in the male:

- coronal sulcus
- glans penis
- inner surface of prepuce
- frenum
- meatus
- anal area
- rectum
- oropharynx
- perineum (often wrongly diagnosed as a fissure)

less commonly:

- lips
- tonsils
- fingers
- buttocks
- nipples

and in women:

- vulva
- labia
- cervix (occasionally)

After the chancre has healed, there may be a latent phase or the second-. ary stage may start immediately.

Secondary stage

This heralds the onset of disseminated disease with a red, non-irritating, maculo-papular rash and generalized painless lymphadenopathy. The rash often covers the trunk and limbs and may be especially marked on the face, palms and soles. Other symptoms may be:

- low-grade fever
- headache
- malaise

- pain in muscles and joints
- occasional patchy alopecia
- sore throat with mucous patches on the tonsils and snail-track ulcers of the fauces

On moist regions of the body – the perineum, external female genitalia and perianal area – moist skin lesions may develop teeming with treponemes. These are known as 'condylomata lata' and look like flat warts. On account of the vast numbers of treponemes present, they are highly infectious.

All evidence of early syphilis disappears in time and sometimes this remission is permanent. Late manifestations of syphilis may occur which involve virtually all the tissues of the body.

Late syphilis

Tertiary syphilis can cause destruction of organs and tissue. The tissues most commonly involved are:

- skin
- mucous membranes
- subcutaneous and submucous tissues
- bones
- joints
- ligaments

Gummas may form in these tissues. These are localized single or multiple lesions and are classed as granulomas. Neurosyphilis and cardiovascular syphilis are the eventual result of untreated syphilis.

Congenital syphilis

Syphilis contracted *in utero* can cause death of the foetus, multi-organ malformations or latent infections. Infants may be born without any sign of disease but later develop rhinitis, rash, bony destruction and cardiovascular symptoms.

Diagnosis

Ulcers can usually clearly be seen on clinical examination of the genital area. This is sometimes performed by nurses who must be competent to clearly recognize ulcers and their significance. In the case of syphilis, ulceration can occur on other parts of the body and could be missed in the absence of careful questioning of the patient and close examination of the skin and mouth.

Treponema pallidum cannot be seen using simple stains, so dark-ground microscopy is used for identification.

Dark-ground microscopy

The lesion, sore, papule or mucous patch should be scraped and the serum mounted on a slide with a cover slip. This is then immediately observed under dark-field microscopy with a 40–100× objective. If present, the spirochetes appear silvery against the dark background. They move in a characteristic way, opening and closing their coil and bending often to an acute angle. If the first sample is negative the patient may be asked to return twice more for further sampling.

Culture is generally unsuccessful. Examination of samples from oral lesions is unhelpful as the oral spirochetes present in the normal flora cause confusion.

Immunofluorescent staining

The specimen is placed on a slide and fixed with acetone. It is examined using a fluorescein-labelled monoclonal antibody. Being a more complex procedure, this is not usually performed in GUM clinics.

Serology

VDRL (Venereal Disease Research Laboratory) test and RPR (rapid plasma reagin)

These are non-treponemal antibody tests which measure a non-specific gamma globulin known as 'reagin'. This is thought to be an auto-antibody produced against host tissues damaged by treponemes. Both these tests become positive in the early stages of primary infection and remain so until the infection is treated. The tests may take up to a year to become negative after treatment.

FTA-ABS (fluorescent treponemal antibody-absorbed) test

These are treponemal antibody tests which are specific in checking antibodies to the treponeme. The antigen used is dead *T. pallidum*, which is dried and fixed on a slide. The patient's serum is added and if antibody is present it sticks to the treponemes. This is then examined using a fluorescent microscope (Thin, 1982). These tests remain positive longer after treatment, and in those who have had longstanding infection they may remain positive for life.

TPHA (Treponema pallidum haemagglutination) test

At the early untreated infectious stage of syphilis this test may be useful. The antigen in this test is a suspension of red cells with a coat of *T. palli-*

VDRL	TPHA	FTA
Negative	Negative	Negative

No evidence of treponemal disease

VDRL	TPHA	FTA
(1) Negative	Negative	Positive
(2) Positive	Negative	Positive

Early syphilis

VDRL	TPHA	FTA
Negative	Positive	Negative

History of treated syphilis or false positive

VDRL	TPHA	FTA
Negative	Positive	Positive

Treated syphilis

VDRL	TPHA	FTA
Positive	Negative	Negative

Possible false positive

Figure 6.1 General interpretation of serological tests for syphilis.

dum. Once the serum is added haemagglutination occurs if syphilis is present.To aid diagnosis a general interpretation of serological tests for syphilis is useful – shown in Figure 6.1. It is also important to note that a small number of individuals with HIV infection who acquire syphilis may fail to produce anti-treponemal antibodies and may therefore remain undiagnosed. A screen for other sexually transmitted infections is advisable.

Treatment

The treatment of choice for syphilis is procaine penicillin. In the primary or secondary stage, intramuscular injections of 600,000 units for 12–20 days is found to be most effective, giving a cure rate of 95% (Csonka and Oates, 1990). If there is a history of penicillin allergy the following may be used:

- Oxytetracycline 500 mg four times daily for 30 days.
- Doxycycline 200 mg twice daily for 21 days.
- Azithromycin also has potential for the treatment of syphilis for those allergic to penicillin. The recommended dosage would be 500 mg daily for 10 days (Mashkilleyson *et al.*, 1996).

Two types of adverse reaction to treatment have been noted:

1. The Jarisch–Herxheimer reaction resulting from the massive destruction of the treponemes by initial doses of antibiotic (Goldmeier and Hay, 1993). The symptoms of this include:

- flu-like signs
- rapid heartbeat
- fever
- chills
- headache
- sore throat
- increased redness of the skin

Patients are advised that this reaction will occur only after the first treatment and not after subsequent injections or oral intake of the antibiotics. A steroid preparation may be given to reduce the reaction.

2. An immediate reaction after the injection manifesting in:

- tachycardia
- hyperventilation
- vomiting
- hysteria
- cardiac collapse on occasion; no recorded fatalities

This reaction is observed to pass spontaneously (Csonka and Oates, 1990).

If procaine penicillin is required the nursing staff administer the injections on a daily basis. The long course of treatment enables the nurse and patient to build rapport. This relationship provides opportunities for the nurse to offer advice and information about the infection and to reinforce the importance of preventing further infections.

Treatment is not normally advised for the contacts of those treated for syphilis unless the existence of the infection is confirmed.

Follow-up

Follow-up is essential and includes clinical examination and repeat serology tests to ensure the infection has been eradicated. Serology should be repeated:

- monthly for three months after starting treatment
- three-monthly until a year after starting treatment
- at 18 months after starting treatment
- at two years after starting treatment

Contact tracing is important. Partners of those infected with syphilis must be examined and treated if appropriate in order to prevent further spread.

Congenital syphilis is rare in this country as all pregnant women are tested for syphilis. If positive serology is found in pregnancy the mother is treated and followed up in the normal way.

Information and advice about safe sex is important for the prevention of reinfection. In addition to this it has been confirmed that genital ulcer disease, including syphilis, can increase susceptibility to infections such as HIV by damaging the mucosal epithelium, which allows easy access into the body (Greenblatt, Lukehart and Plummer, 1991). This is particularly important in developing countries where access to GU services and condoms are limited. Thus control of genital ulcer disease is important in the control of HIV. This fact must be acknowledged and discussed with each individual as appropriate.

CHANCROID

Chancroid manifests as a soft ulcer found principally in the genital area. It is common in developing countries.

Microbiology

Chancroid is caused by a small Gram-negative bacillus called *Haemophilus ducreyi*. It has an incubation period of approximately one week.

Epidemiology

In the United Kingdom chancroid is rare and is classified as a tropical disease. Data on this infection are collected along with those on lymphogranuloma venereum and granuloma inguinale, so it is difficult to establish how many cases of each have been reported. In England in 1984 the collective reported cases of all three infections was 100, declining to 62 in 1994 (Department of Health, 1995).

Transmission

Chancroid is transmitted by direct sexual contact. It is more common in men, especially those who are uncircumcised.

Signs and symptoms

The main signs of chancroid are sores on the genitals, which may be multiple, painful and sometimes foul smelling. The ulcer has been described as a 'soft' chancre as opposed to the 'hard' chancre of syphilis. There is often pain and tenderness in the inguinal glands.

Diagnosis

Again, the recognition of genital ulceration and its significance is important.

Microscopy

Scrapings from the ulcer may be viewed under the microscope but this method lacks sensitivity.

Culture

This is possible but *H. ducreyi* is notoriously difficult to culture. Optimum conditions for growth are 33–34°C in 5% carbon dioxide at high humidity. Growth can be observed after 48–72 hours' incubation.

Serology

It is important to exclude syphilis by serology testing. Screening for other sexually transmitted infections is also advisable.

Treatment

Usually tetracyclines, erythromycin or cephalosporins.

Follow-up

This is important to ensure that the ulcers have healed and the lymphadenopathy is resolving. Contact tracing is also necessary in order to halt the spread of the infection. This can be very difficult if the infection was contracted abroad; therefore safer sex advice is essential to prevent further spread and reinfection. The significance of genital ulceration in the transmission of other infections such as HIV must be acknowledged and discussed with the individual as appropriate.

GRANULOMA INGUINALE

This is an uncommon, moderately contagious, almost chronic disease involving skin, subcutaneous tissue and lymphatic glands. It is also known as Donovanosis.

Microbiology

Granuloma inguinale is caused by the Donovan body, a minute protozoan that is recoverable from the lesions. It mainly occurs in the tropics. Although the incubation period is uncertain, it is on average 4–6 weeks.

Transmission

It is usually sexually transmitted.

Signs and symptoms

The early lesion is a papule, vesicle or nodule which erodes and becomes an ulcer with a red granular base. It often presents as a red, smooth mass of granulation tissue on the prepuce or vulva. The margins of the lesion are not well defined and may bleed easily but are not painful. They do not heal quickly, their border having a rolled edge. The ulcerative process may be static for years and scarring occurs. The inguinal swelling in this disease is a subcutaneous granuloma, not an adenitis.

Diagnosis

This is confirmed by taking a scraping from the lesion on to a slide and staining it by Giemsa's method. The coccal-like organism can be observed, surrounded by a halo of encapsulation lying within epithelial cells.

Treatment

The drugs of choice are:

- co-trimoxazole
- tetracyclines
- erythromycin

LYMPHOGRANULOMA VENEREUM

This disease is widespread throughout the world, although most common in tropical countries.

Microbiology

Lymphogranuloma venereum is caused by *Chlamydia trachomatis* (see Chapter 8). The incubation period is 1–4 weeks.

Transmission

It is usually sexually transmitted.

Signs and symptoms

The organism spreads via the lymph glands and may result locally in bubo formation, ulceration and elephantitis. A primary lesion is not always seen, but if present consists of a minute, painless papule or vesicle. If untreated the bubo is recognized up to a month later and is firm and elongated. Irregular areas of softening develop, followed by suppuration and sometimes by the formation of fistulae. Lymphatic blockage may cause elephantitis. A sore on the penis results in inguinal adenitis, in the vagina a pelvi-rectal adenitis, and in the ano-rectal region a peri-rectal adenitis. The primary lesion often heals spontaneously but chronic ulceration can occur locally.

Diagnosis

This can be made by specific antibody complement fixation tests. Formerly a skin test was used.

Treatment

Oral tetracycline 250 mg six-hourly for ten days is the drug of choice. Sulphonamides and erythromycin can also prove effective.

GLOSSARY

Adenitis	Inflammation of a lymph node or any gland
Alopecia	Baldness
Bubo	A swelling in the groin or armpit from enlargement of lymph nodes as a result of infection
Elephantitis	Enormous enlargement of genitalia or a limb, caused by obstruction of lymph drainage
Fauces	The space at the back of the mouth and pharynx under the soft palate and between the soft palatine arches
Fistulae	Abnormal communications between any part of the interior of the body and skin surface or between two internal organs
Gamma globulin	A protein, one of the five classes of immunoglobulins
Granulation tissue	Tissue that forms on the surface of a wound during healing

Granuloma	A localized mass of granulation tissue forming a nodule
Haemagglutination	Clumping together of red blood cells
Lymphadenopathy	Any disease process affecting a lymph node
Monoclonal antibodies	Antibodies produced by hybrid B lymphocyte tumours
Protozoan	A single-celled microscopic organism
Serology	Investigation of blood serum, especially noting its antibody content
Subcutaneous	Under the skin
Suppuration	The production or discharge of pus

REFERENCES

Chang, S.N., Chung, K.-Y., Lee, M.-G., and Lee, J.B. (1995) Seroconversion of the serological tests for syphilis in the newborns born to treated syphilitic mothers. *Genitouriary Medicine*, **71**(2), 68–70.

Csonka, G.W. and Oates, J.K. (eds) (1990) *Sexually Transmitted Diseases: A Textbook of Genitourinary Medicine*, Baillière Tindall, London.

Department of Health (1995) *Statistical Bulletin: Sexually Transmitted Diseases, England 1994*, Bulletin 1995/16

Goldmeier, D. and Hay, P. (1993) A review and update on adult syphilis, with particular reference to its treatment. *International Journal of STD & AIDS*, **4**(2), 70–82.

Greenblatt R.M., Lukehart, S.A. and Plummer, F.A. (1991) Genital ulceration as a risk factor for human immunodeficiency virus infection. *AIDS*, **2**, 47–50

Mashkilleyson, A.L., Gomberg, M.A., Mashkilleyson, N. and Kutin, S.A. (1996) Treatment of syphilis with azithromycin. *International Journal of STD & AIDS*, **7**(Supp 1), 13–16.

Thin, R.N. (1982) *Lecture Notes on Sexually Transmitted Diseases*, Blackwell Scientific Publications, Oxford.

Gonorrhoea

7

OBJECTIVES

1. To describe the microbiology of *Neisseria gonorrhoeae*.
2. To recognize the main signs and symptoms of gonococcal infection.
3. To explain the consequences of untreated gonococcal infection.
4. To identify the main techniques used for diagnosing gonorrhoea.
5. To list the common treatment regimes for gonorrhoea.
6. To explain the follow-up and contact tracing of gonococcal infections.

SUMMARY

Neisseria gonorrhoeae is a common sexually transmitted infection, which if left untreated can cause serious complications. Once diagnosed it is easily treated with antibiotics but the risk of reinfection is high without good follow-up procedures and contact tracing. It is an ancient infection, the history of which is described in Chapter 1.

This chapter describes the microbiology, transmission, symptomology, diagnosis and treatment of gonorrhoea.

EPIDEMIOLOGY

In the United Kingdom the incidence of gonorrhoea reached its peak in the 1970s and early 1980s with 50,000 reported cases a year. In 1994 the number of new cases was 11,574, the drop in incidence attributed to safer sex campaigns for the prevention of HIV. This down trend now appears to have halted. The total number of new cases in 1994 includes 16% who were treated epidemiologically (Department of Health, 1995). The epidemiology of gonorrhoea is examined more closely in Chapter 3.

MICROBIOLOGY

Gonorrhoea is caused by *Neisseria gonorrhoeae*, a Gram-negative, intra-cellular diplococcus. The bacteria are bean shaped and appear in pairs. They have a loose capsule and attach to the mucosal epithelium by hair-like appendages called pili. They grow optimally at 35–37°C in a 5% carbon dioxide atmosphere and do not survive long outside the body. Once inside the body the organism produces endotoxins causing tissue destruction and inflammation. The incubation period is usually 2–7 days.

Strains of gonorrhoea resistant to penicillin were noted in the 1970s (Phillips, 1976), especially in the Far East (Seghal and Srivastva, 1987). These strains have the ability to produce penicillinase, leading to part or total resistance to penicillin. Despite fears that these strains of gonorrhoea would become endemic in the United Kingdom, they remain only a small percentage of all strains seen. These strains appeared to originate in Africa and South East Asia but now the Caribbean is the most usual source (Sherrard and Barlow, 1993). Other strains of gonococci have been identified which appear to be resistant to other antibiotics.

TRANSMISSION

Gonorrhoea is sexually transmitted, which includes via close genital contact. Through oral and anal sex it can also affect the throat and anal canal. The risk of infection for women after one exposure to an infected man is 60–90% and for men after one exposure to an infected woman 20–50% (Sherrard and Bingham, 1995).

Babies born to mothers with gonorrhoea can acquire eye or vulval infections on their way though the birth canal.

SIGNS AND SYMPTOMS

Gonococci attack mucous membranes and columnar epithelium in parti-cular, causing an inflammatory reaction and a violent polymorphonuclear response.

Men

The usual first sign of gonococcal infection in men is a purulent yellow urethral discharge accompanied by burning and discomfort on passing urine. The meatus may also be reddened and tender. There is often a history of unprotected intercourse in the previous week. Other symptoms can include:

- rectal discharge and soreness
- on proctoscopy, reddened appearance of rectal mucosa
- sore throat

A small proportion of men experience no symptoms.

Women

In women there are frequently no symptoms at all. If symptoms are present they consist of:

- abnormal vaginal discharge
- lower abdominal pain
- dysuria

Complications

These are less frequent in men, owing to the early presence of symptoms, but could be:

- penile oedema
- peri-urethral abscess
- epididymitis
- prostatitis
- urethral stricture (rare)

Complications are more frequent in women as a direct result of the absence or mildness of symptoms. Complications may include:

- pelvic inflammatory disease (see Chapter 10)
- peritonitis
- endometritis
- bartholinitis
- peri-hepatitis (Fitz-Hugh-Curtis syndrome)

The diagnosis and treatment of gonorrhoea in pregnant women is particularly important as there is some suggestion that the presence of gonococcus may increase the risk of premature birth or a low birthweight baby (Donders *et al.*, 1993)

Disseminated gonococcal infection is the spread of gonorrhoea throughout the bloodstream. This is rare but in both sexes can lead to:

- fever
- arthralgias
- arthritis
- pustular rash

If there are no genital symptoms this diagnosis can be missed.

Children

If a woman is infected at the time of parturition the baby's eyes may become contaminated with gonococci, giving rise to a condition known as 'ophthalmia neonatorum'. If treated promptly this can be eradicated with no lasting complications. However, if left it can lead to corneal ulceration and blindness. Oropharyngeal infection may also be found in a proportion of these children.

Urethral gonococcal infection in boys is indicative of sexual activity, but vulvo-vaginal symptoms in girls can arise from non-sexual contact with a parent. In prepubertal children, sexual abuse must be considered if gonorrhoea is diagnosed.

A similar organism, *Neisseria meningitidis*, which can asymptomatically colonize the nasopharynx, rarely causes similar urethral symptoms as gonorrhoea. It is appropriate to treat this in the same way until the identity of the organism is clear.

DIAGNOSIS

Good quality specimens must be collected for the accurate diagnosis of gonorrhoea.

Microscopy

In men the prepuce is retracted and a plastic loop is inserted 1–2 cm inside the urethra and gently scraped to collect secretions. The patient should not have passed urine less than two hours before the examination. In women specimens are taken in a similar way from the endocervix and urethra. The specimens are then smeared onto a glass slide and stained using the Gram staining method.

High-powered magnification (× 1000) is used to identify polymorphonuclear leucocytes containing the intracellular Gram-negative diplococci. This procedure is usually carried out by a nurse who is highly skilled in the identification of these bacteria.

National standards for the immediate diagnosis of gonorrhoea by microscopy are (Fitzgerald et al., 1996):

- 40% of female specimens (urethral, endocervical)
- 90% of male specimens (urethral).

Culture

Each time a specimen is smeared on to a slide a culture plate is also inoculated. Although in men the diagnosis is usually made using microscopy, this is more difficult in women and cultures are essential to confirm the diagnosis (Mardh and Danielsson, 1990). In addition samples from the rectum and pharynx are cultured. It is recommended that pharyngeal cultures are taken from all individuals with a possible exposure to gonorrhoea regardless of whether they have a history of oral sex (Barlow, 1997). Microscopy is difficult with such specimens, due to contamination by other organisms.

The culture plates must be prewarmed and inoculated immediately; the gonococci are fragile and need optimum conditions for growth. The plates must then be incubated at between 35 and 37°C and kept in an atmosphere of 5% carbon dioxide. If laboratory facilities are unavailable, Stuart's transport medium may be used. The culture plates are then examined in the laboratory after 24 and 48 hours' incubation. If suspect colonies are observed, various tests are performed to confirm the identity of the organism.

The antibiotic sensitivities of the organism should be established. This is particularly important in the case of gonorrhoea as penicillin-resistant strains must be identified to ensure effective treatment. It is important to screen for other sexually transmitted infections at this time.

TREATMENT

Gonococci are sensitive to a wide range of antibiotics although penicillin has been the drug of choice for many years. A single dose treatment is ideal to ensure patient compliance. The usual regimes are:

- ampicillin 2–3.5 g and probenecid 1 g orally stat dose
- ciprofloxacin 250–500 mg orally stat dose
- spectinomycin 2 g intramuscular injection stat dose
- amoxycillin 3 g and 1 g probenecid orally
- ofloxacin 400 mg orally
- norfloxacin 800 mg orally
- azithromycin 1–2g orally

Disseminated gonorrhoea requires a longer course of treatment

The treatment chosen should be expected to eradicate 95% of gonococcal infections. In pharyngeal gonorrhoea the expected eradication rate is 90%. Epidemiological treatment may be given to the contacts of people known to have gonorrhoea; this is a decision taken by the clinician after considering each individual case. Such treatment is often given when microscopic detection may be difficult, e.g. in the cervix, rectum or pharynx due to contamination by other organisms.

It has been suggested that if gonococcal infections are suspected to have been acquired in Africa, South East Asia or the Caribbean, then appropriate treatment for penicillin-resistant organisms should be administered before the antibiotic sensitivity results are available (Sherrard and Barlow, 1993).

FOLLOW-UP

A diagnosis of gonorrhoea requires a strict regime of follow-up to prevent reinfection and further spread of the infection (Fitzgerald and Bedford, 1996). It is recommended that at least one but preferably two follow-up swab tests are performed. This involves retesting the infected sites and also a set of throat and rectal swabs. If these were the initial sites of infection, swabs must be taken on at least one more occasion after treatment. The tests of cure should be approximately three and ten days after treatment and performed even when epidemiological treatment has been administered. It is usually the nurse's role to manage this follow-up regime, which requires assessment, communication and practical skills (see Chapter 17).

Fitzgerald and colleagues (1996) produced standards for contact tracing in gonorrhoea, to be followed by all GUM clinics in the United Kingdom. Key points were:

- All patients with gonorrhoea should be seen by a health adviser at the time of treatment.
- All patients with gonorrhoea should discuss partner notification at the time of treatment.
- Each clinic should have an effective recall system for those with untreated infection or who fail to arrive for follow-up.
- Accurate and concise documentation of contact tracing.
- Use of contact slips should be encouraged.

Health education and safer sex advice is essential for preventing reinfection with gonorrhoea. It is well documented that there is a cohort of patients who acquire repeated infections of gonorrhoea; these patients are often male, single and black. The challenge for GUM clinics is to target these individuals to negotiate condom use and reduction in the number of partners, taking account of social and cultural factors (Sherrard and Barlow, 1996).

In many GUM clinics it is the role of the health adviser to give advice and information to those with or at risk of a sexually transmitted infection. They also deal with contact tracing. In some clinics these interventions are carried out by multi-skilled nurses who have taken on the duties elsewhere carried out by a health adviser. When both disciplines of staff are present in a larger multidisciplinary team the information given must be consistent and the nurse and health adviser should work together to reinforce safer sex advice and to formulate a joint prevention strategy. Such joint working is essential when dealing with infections such as gonorrhoea where there is a high reinfection rate. It is common for nurses to underutilize their knowledge by referring patients to the health adviser before giving any information or advice. The importance of repetition and reinforcement of information is pertinent here and should be recognized as part of the nurse's role.

The diagnosis and follow-up of gonorrhoea is often managed by nurses and this practice should be regularly audited in order to evaluate and improve services. The National Standards for the Management of Gonorrhoea (Fitzgerald and Bedford, 1996) provide an excellent basis from which to audit service provision. The management of gonorrhoea, for example, is often audited by medical staff. This will include the success of diagnostic methods and follow-up strategies, usually carried out by nurses. Nurses must become more involved in audit so they can develop their practice and demand ownership and recognition of their skills.

GLOSSARY

Arthralgias	Pains in the joints
Bartholinitis	Inflammation, sometimes with abscess formation, in the Bartholin's glands
Diplococcus	Cocci that occur in pairs
Endometritis	Inflammation of the endometrium
Epidemiological (treatment)	Where treatment is administered to contacts of proven individuals even though the contacts' diagnosis has not been confirmed
Epididymitis	Inflammation of the epididymus
Peri-hepatitis	Inflammation of the membranes surrounding the liver
Peritonitis	Inflammation of the perineum
Prostatitis	Inflammation of the prostate gland

REFERENCES

Barlow, D. (1997) The diagnosis of oropharyngeal gonorrhoea. *Genitourinary Medicine*, **73**(1), 16–17.
Department of Health (1995) *Statistical Bulletin: Sexually Transmitted Diseases,*

England 1994, Bulletin 1995/16.

Donders, G.G.G., Desmyter, J., De Wet, D.H. and Van Assche, F.A. (1993) The association of gonorrhoea and syphilis with premature birth and low birthweight. *Genitourinary Medicine*, **69**(2), 98–101.

Fitzgerald, M. and Bedford, C. (1996) National standards for the management of gonorrhoea. *International Journal of STD and AIDS*, **7**(4), 298–301.

Fitzgerald, M., Thirlby, D., Bell, G. and Bedford, C. (1996) National standards for contact tracing in gonorrhoea. *International Journal of STD and AIDS*, **7**(4), 301.

Mardh, P.-A. and Danielsson, D. (1990) *Neisseria gonorrhoeae, in Sexually Transmitted Infections*, 2nd edn (eds K.K. Holmes, P.-A. Mardh, P.F. Sparling and P.J. Wiesner), McGraw-Hill. New York.

Murray, P.R., Drew, W.L., Kobayashi, G.S. and Thompson, J.H. (1990) *Medical Microbiology*, Wolfe, USA.

Phillips, I. (1976) Beta-lactamase producing penicillin resistant gonococcus. *Lancet*, **2**, 656.

Seghal, V.N. and Srivastva, G. (1987) Gonorrhoea and the story of resistant *Neisseria gonorrhoeae*. *International Journal of Dermatology*, **26**, 206–13.

Sherrard, J. and Barlow, D. (1993) PPNG at St Thomas' Hospital – a changing provenance. *International Journal of STD and AIDS*, **4**(6), 330–2.

Sherrard, J. and Barlow, D. (1996) Men with repeated episodes of gonorrhoea 1990–1992. *International Journal of STD and AIDS*, **7**(4), 281–3.

Sherrard, J. and Bingham, J.S. (1995) Gonorrhoea now. *International Journal of STD and AIDS*, **6**(3), 162–6.

Chlamydial infection 8

OBJECTIVES

1. To describe the microbiology of *Chlamydia trachomatis*.
2. To recognize the main symptoms of chlamydia infection in both men and women.
3. To explain the consequences of untreated chlamydia infection for men, women and the newborn.
4. To identify the main techniques used to diagnose chlamydia infection.
5. To list the treatment regimes for chlamydia infection.
6. To explain the importance of follow-up and contact tracing in cases of chlamydia infection.

SUMMARY

Chlamydia trachomatis is one of the most common sexually transmitted organisms. Despite this, however, there appears to be an ignorance surrounding it not found with more familiar infections such as gonorrhoea, which is often seen as much more serious. The consequences of chlamydia can be serious, although once detected it is easily destroyed by antibiotics. This chapter will describe the microbiology, transmission, symptomology, diagnosis and treatment of *Chlamydia trachomatis* infection.

EPIDEMIOLOGY

Chlamydia is one of the most common sexually transmitted diseases in England (Department of Health, 1995). It is suspected that the reported cases represent only a fraction of the true number of infections. Cases of chlamydia identified in other clinics and GP surgeries may go unreported, making it difficult to establish accurate trends.

The incidence of chlamydia was first recorded separately in 1989. In GUM clinics in England the number of new cases of chlamydia remained steady between 33,000 and 37,000 in the years 1989 to 1994, with slightly more reported cases in women, 19,120 in 1994.

The majority of identified cases are of postpubertal uncomplicated chlamydia, 27,574 cases in 1994. Most of the remainder comprise epidemiological treatment of chlamydia, where treatment is given to contacts of patients with a diagnosis of chlamydia without their own diagnosis having been confirmed. This accounts for 23% of cases in 1994, compared to 15% in 1989. Of the total number of new cases of postpubertal uncomplicated chlamydia reported in 1994 only 2% were estimated as having been homosexually acquired.

Chlamydia is often found in conjunction with other sexually transmitted infections such as gonorrhoea.

MICROBIOLOGY

The classification of *Chlamydia trachomatis* is open to debate. It is neither a true bacterium nor a virus but appears to show characteristics of both. It has inner and outer membranes with a rigid cell wall and contains many structures similar to those of Gram-negative bacteria. Nevertheless, like a virus, it relies on a host cell for energy and reproduction, which is achieved by binary fission. Although non-motile and without pili there are surface projections which allow uptake of nutrients from the host cells. This organism displays a unique growth cycle featuring the following two forms of chlamydiae (see Figure 8.1).

Elementary body

This is the infectious form and is extracellular. The growth cycle begins with this form. The elementary body attaches itself to the host cell and then penetrates it. After 6–8 hours inside, it becomes metabolically active and is then termed the 'reticulate body'.

Reticulate body

The reticulate bodies, which are non-infectious, reproduce by binary fission 8–24 hours after infection. They are then termed 'inclusion bodies'. These inclusion bodies are evident under immunofluorescence for diagnosis of chlamydia. After 18–24 hours the reticulate bodies become elementary bodies again and are released from the cell.

Chlamydia trachomatis appears to infect only non-ciliated, columnar or

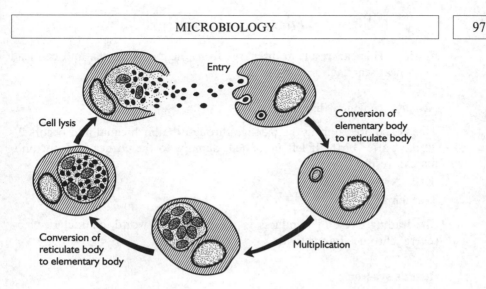

Figure 8.1 The life cycle of *Chlamydia trachomatis*

cuboidal epithelium. This explains its preference for certain surfaces of the body:

- conjunctiva
- endocervix
- urethra
- rectum
- endometrium
- uterine tubes

Chlamydia trachomatis is divided into three biovars, the two human strains being:

- lymphogranuloma venereum
- trachoma

Chlamydia trachomatis is the cause of a wide range of diseases:

Urogenital infections

In men this infectious agent is responsible for a high proportion of cases of non-specific urethritis. It is also one of the most common and serious causes of pelvic inflammatory disease in women (see Chapter 10).

Adult inclusion conjunctivitis

Although this is usually associated with genital infection, auto-innoculation and oral–genital contact are believed to be the main routes of transmission. This can result in discharge from the eye, keratitis, and can lead to corneal scarring.

Neonatal conjunctivitis

This is acquired during the passage through the birth canal and occurs 2–30 days after birth. If left untreated, damage to the cornea and pneumonia can result.

Trachoma

The leading cause of blindness in the developing world, characterized by severe, chronic conjunctivitis.

Reiter's syndrome

A complex disease process, in some cases believed to be triggered by a genital infection with *Chlamydia trachomatis* and characterized by urethritis, conjunctivitis, polyarthritis and mucocutaneous lesions. The condition usually occurs in young white males.

TRANSMISSION

Urogenital infections of *Chlamydia trachomatis* are sexually transmitted, the bacteria gaining access through minute abrasions in the mucous membrane. Certain risk factors for susceptibility to chlamydia infection are suggested (Fish *et al.*, 1989), including:

- Multiple sexual partners, allowing more opportunity for transmission of the organism.
- The presence of cervical ectopy: the transitional zone of the cervix protrudes from the endocervical canal, leaving these more vulnerable cells more open to infection.
- Use of oral contraceptives, which can induce ectopy. Moreover, as the cells of the transitional zone are more accessible when ectopy is present, a higher detection rate for chlamydia may occur. The link between oral contraceptives and chlamydia is far from proven and further research is necessary (Cottingham and Hunter, 1992).
- Termination of pregnancy: there appears to be a higher incidence of chlamydia in women attending for this procedure.

It should be noted that certain groups of women – those using oral contraception and those attending for termination of pregnancy – have been studied more closely than others. This may account for the apparent high incidence of chlamydia infection in these groups.

It is for some of the reasons above that the incidence of chlamydia infection is higher in people under 25 (Department of Health, 1995). It has been observed that sexually active teenage girls are particularly at risk of chlamydia infection. Suggested predisposing factors in this group are (Rahm, Odlind and Pettersson, 1991):

- a new sexual partner
- previous chlamydia infection
- smoking

Orogenital transmission of chlamydia can occur. However, the role of the oropharynx as a reservoir of infection is uncertain. In this area there are rarely any symptoms or physical signs on examination and the organism is difficult to isolate.

It has been suggested from a study of prostitutes in Cameroon that chlamydia may be a co-factor in the transmission of HIV. Chlamydia increases the friability of the cells of the cervix, leaving them more susceptible to infection with HIV (Kaptue *et al.*, 1991). More research is needed to confirm these findings.

SIGNS AND SYMPTOMS

Women

Chlamydia trachomatis infection of the genital tract is often asymptomatic in women. Nevertheless the infection can still spread and if untreated can cause:

- Cervicitis. The cervix may appear swollen and bleed when touched.
- Endometritis.
- Urethritis. This can occur without cervicitis.
- Bartholinitis.
- Peri-hepatitis, also known as Fitz-Hugh-Curtis syndrome. The organism spreads from the pelvis to the liver via the lymphatic system or the peritoneum, causing inflammation and some exudate. Pain in the upper right quadrant of the abdomen may be experienced, often accompanied by lower abdominal pain due to pelvic inflammatory disease.
- Proctitis. Although chlamydia may be present in the rectum, usually through contamination from the vagina, there may be no symptoms. Blood in the stools is often the only sign.
- Salpingitis and tubal scarring. This is usually by the direct route through the cervix, facilitated by sexual intercourse, gynaecological procedures or previous organ damage. In addition, chlamydia can be detected in the uterine tubes without being isolated on the cervix.

If chlamydia infection is left untreated, pelvic inflammatory disease (PID) may develop, the long-term consequences of which could be:

- recurrent pain
- increased chance of ectopic pregnancy
- impaired fertility

PID is discussed in greater detail in Chapter 10.

Consequences for the fetus and the newborn

Chlamydia has been implicated in:

- ectopic pregnancy
- premature membrane rupture
- spontaneous abortion

In the newborn, chlamydia can manifest itself in serious ways:

- conjunctivitis
- pneumonia
- otitis media

Men

Generally *Chlamydia trachomatis* infections in men are symptomatic, causing a non-specific urethritis (NSU). Chlamydia is not the only cause of urethritis; other organisms may also be responsible and are discussed in Chapter 9.

Chlamydia is often associated with gonorrhoea and is also one of the main causes of post-gonococcal urethritis. The chlamydia continue to multiply during the treatment for gonorrhoea.

The main symptoms of NSU caused by chlamydia are:

- urethral discharge, usually clear or white
- pain on passing urine
- epididymo-orchitis
- testicular pain
- proctitis

As mentioned previously, in some cases of untreated NSU caused by chlamydia a reactive arthritis may occur.

DIAGNOSIS

Routine screening for *Chlamydia trachomatis* is carried out in GUM clinics. This is recommended, as it is recognized that many men and women have no clinical signs of infection at the time of examination. Diagnosis of chlamydia in both men and women is more complex than that of other infections such as gonorrhoea. While gonorrhoea can be diagnosed on immediate microscopic inspection of a urethral or cervical specimen, the detection of chlamydia is far more complex.

Women

A swab is taken from the endocervix and/or urethra and sent to the laboratory for analysis. A cotton-tipped swab is usually used to collect the endocervical specimen. Other methods of specimen collection have also been found effective, such as the cytobrush (Szarewski *et al.*, 1989). To avoid trauma to the cervix the cytobrush is not recommended for use in pregnancy.

Recent research has shown that chlamydia can also be isolated from first void urine samples (Svensson, Mares and Olsson, 1991). This method may be useful in settings where invasive swabbing of all women for chlamydia is difficult, e.g. GP surgeries. It must be borne in mind that chlamydia present in the cervix alone will not be detected by this method.

On examination of a Gram stained cervical slide, polymorphonuclear leucocytes may be seen; however, at this stage it is impossible to attribute these to chlamydia as so many other factors are involved. The number of leucocytes seen could be due to:

- the influence of the menstrual cycle
- oral contraception
- intrauterine contraceptive device
- sexual activity
- the presence of other infections, e.g. gonorrhoea

Men

Swabs are taken from the urethra and for gay men from the rectum. These are then sent to the laboratory for analysis.

As with women, studies have suggested that chlamydia can be detected in the urine using various laboratory methods and these should provide a non-invasive alternative for chlamydia diagnosis. It does appear that this method could be as successful as urethral swabbing, particularly in men who had not held their urine for more than three hours before urethral sampling (Hay *et al.*, 1991). However, it is accepted that urethral swabbing still remains the superior method of specimen collection (Matthew, 1993). In settings where chlamydia culture is not available, the first catch urine sampling technique using an enzyme immunoassay may still be of value.

In men NSU can be diagnosed quickly by microscopic examination of a Gram stained smear of urethral discharge. This can be collected from a urethral swab or from a thread in a urine sample. The detection of a significant number of polymorphonuclear leucocytes in the absence of gonococcus suggests NSU. A urethral swab for chlamydia is also taken. However, treatment is given on the assumption that chlamydia is the cause.

It is important to emphasize that symptomatic infections with *Chlamydia trachomatis* yield more organisms on culture than do asymptomatic infections. As this organism is dependent on host cells for energy and replication it cannot be grown artificially. A tissue culture is necessary to detect the organism, a characteristic that demonstrates its relationship to viruses.

Chlamydia trachomatis can be detected in various ways:

Cell culture

After 48–72 hours the culture is stained with iodine or an immunofluorescent stain and microscopically examined. This method is highly sensitive but is complicated and expensive. In addition the specimen must be of good quality, maintained at 4°C and transported to the laboratory promptly to ensure that the cells remain viable. However, the method does remain the gold standard for the detection of chlamydia.

Direct antigen detection in clinical specimens

This can be done by enzyme-linked immunosorbent assay (ELISA). For symptomatic women the sensitivity is greater than 90% but much lower in men and asymptomatic women. False positives are not uncommon. This test is generally used for screening purposes.

Immunofluorescent techniques

These can also be used for direct antigen testing.

Serological testing

The value of this method is limited because it is as yet impossible to differentiate between past and current infection.

Clearview

The 'Clearview Chlamydia' test for rapid detection of chlamydia from cervical specimens has recently been evaluated. Although further work is necessary, this method may prove valuable where rapid results are needed or access to laboratory facilities is limited (Young *et al.*, 1991). This method might be particularly useful in the general practice setting because nurses would be able to perform chlamydia testing without the need for on-site laboratory facilities. This type of test enables the identification and treatment of many cases of women with chlamydia who might otherwise remain undiagnosed and untreated. This is an important development for practice nursing as nurses may be involved in setting up screening programmes in the community.

Polymerase chain reaction (PCR)

This is a recently developed diagnostic test which could greatly increase the sensitivity of detection of *Chlamydia trachomatis*. Recent work has demonstrated good correlation between the PCR and culture results (Martin *et al.*, 1995). Moreover, strict transport conditions for specimens are unnecessary and results can be obtained more quickly. False positive results are a problem but this method may have a future role in chlamydia testing.

Ligase chain reaction (LCR)

This is the most recently developed diagnostic test for chlamydia. Research is currently underway to test its effectiveness. Early studies have suggested that the LCR method will provide a simple, rapid and good alternative test for the detection of chlamydia, although control monitoring will be necessary to avoid false negative results (de Barbeyrac *et al.*, 1997).

TREATMENT

Effective treatment regimes are:

- doxycycline 100 mg twice a day for seven days
- or 200 mg stat, then 100 mg once a day for seven days
- oxytetracycline 500 mg 2–4 times a day for seven days
- erythromycin 500 mg 2–4 times a day for seven days

It is recognized that the lower doses are adequate and may improve compliance. Several studies have been carried out comparing different treatment regimes. It has been shown that cure rates for NSU do not differ significantly whether ofloxacin, doxycycline or erythromycin is used (Kitchen *et al.*, 1990; Moller *et al.*, 1990).

In order to encourage compliance with treatment, work has been carried out on the effectiveness of a 100 mg single dose of azithromycin as opposed to a longer course of other antimicrobials. This has been shown to be as effective (Whatley *et al.*, 1991; Nilsen *et al.*, 1992).

FOLLOW-UP

In many GUM clinics repeat swab tests for chlamydia are performed after treatment. Both the WHO (1989) and the Centers for Disease Control (1989) recommend that this is unnecessary, for two reasons:

- Chlamydial resistance to antimicrobials used in its treatment has never been apparent.
- The re-isolation of chlamydia following treatment is often due to rein-fection rather than treatment failure, because of further exposure to the organism before the end of the course of treatment or before all contacts have been treated.

If reinfection is suspected, a test of cure is indicated, involving taking specimens for chlamydial culture. However, this should be carried out at least a week after the cessation of treatment. Before then antimicrobial activity may inhibit the growth of chlamydia (Radcliffe *et al.*, 1990). Further research has shown that patients should reattend up to 3–4 weeks after treatment, to provide the opportunity for evaluation of contact tracing. Retesting for chlamydia would be indicated only if unprotected intercourse or non-compliance with the treatment had occurred (White *et al.*, 1993).

A follow-up visit should be arranged with a nurse or health adviser after treatment in order to check compliance with treatment and to complete contact tracing in order to minimize the risk of reinfection. If treatment is complete and there has been no chance of reinfection, a further test of cure is unnecessary.

Health education about chlamydia and the ignorance surrounding this infection and its consequences are important, especially if the co-factor link between chlamydia and HIV is proven. Women especially must be educated in how to recognize the signs and symptoms of chlamydia and encouraged to seek advice if an infection is suspected. As many women will remain asymptomatic, education about the mode of transmission of chlamydia and ways of preventing this is essential.

Reinfection with chlamydia is common, indicating the need for raised awareness of the importance of contact tracing and the conse-quences of contacts not being treated. Discussion continues about ways to inform contacts of the infection and of the need for them to be checked. The risk of complications is increased with each subsequent episode of infection, impaired fertility being one of the more serious outcomes.

Some women may believe that a cervical smear test is also tested for infections such as chlamydia and it must be made clear that other tests are necessary if accurate diagnoses are to be made. Sometimes in GP surgeries or family planning clinics the correct testing equipment is not available. The GUM clinic is the ideal place to have examination and investigations performed, as the necessary equipment and laboratory support is on-site. Rapid testing kits are currently being developed to make it easier for chlamydia testing to be carried out where laboratory facilities are not immediately available.

GLOSSARY

Bartholinitis	Inflammation, sometimes with abscess formation, in the Bartholin's glands
Endometritis	Inflammation of the endometrium
Epididymo-orchitis	Inflammation of the epididymis and testis
Immunoassay	Quantitative estimate of the concentration of various antibodies in blood serum
Immunofluorescence	The detection and identification of antigenic material by observing microscopically the fluorescence of known specific fluorescein-linked antibodies that have become attached to the antigen
Keratitis	Inflammation of the cornea
Mucocutaneous	Pertaining to the mucous membrane and skin
Peri-hepatitis	Inflammation of the membranes surrounding the liver
Polyarthritis	Arthritis affecting many joints
Polymerase chain reaction	A technique for rapidly producing large numbers of copies of any required sequence of DNA
Polymorphonuclear	Having a lobed nucleus of varying lobe number or shape
Proctitis	Inflammation of the rectum
Salpingitis	Inflammation of the uterine tubes

REFERENCES

de Barbeyrac, B., Rodriguez, P., Dutilh, B. *et al.* (1997) Detection of *Chlamydia trachomatis* by ligase chain reaction compared with polymerase chain reaction and cell culture in urogenital specimens. *Genitourinary Medicine*, **71**(6), 382–6.

Centers for Disease Control (1989) Sexually transmitted disease treatment guidelines. MMWR 1989; **38** (S-8), pp. 1–43.

Cottingham, J. and Hunter, D. (1992) *Chlamydia trachomatis* and oral contraceptive use: a quantitative review. *Genitourinary Medicine*, **68**(4), 209–16.

Department of Health (1995) *Statistical Bulletin: Sexually Transmitted Diseases, England 1994*, Bulletin 1995/16.

Fish, A.N.J., Fairweather, D.V.I., Oriel, J.D., Ridgway, G.L. (1989) *Chlamydia trachomatis* infection in a gynaecology clinic population: identification of high risk groups and the value of contact tracing. *European Journal of Obstetrics, Gynaecology and Reproductive Medicine*, **31**, 67–74.

Hay, P.E., Thomas, B.J., Gilchrist, C. *et al.* (1991) The value of urine samples from men with non-gonococcal urethritis for the detection of *Chlamydia trachomatis*. *Genitourinary Medicine*, **67**(2), 124–8.

Kaptue, L., Zekeng, L., Djoumessi, S. *et al.* (1991) HIV and chlamydia infections among prostitutes in Yaounde, Cameroon. *Genitourinary Medicine*, **67**(2), 143–5.

Kitchen, V.S., Donegan, C., Ward, H. *et al.* (1990) Comparison of ofloxacin with doxycycline in the treatment of non-gonoccocal urethritis and cervical chlamydia infection. *Journal of Antimicrobial Chemotherapy*, **26**(Supp.), 99–105.

Martin, J.L., Alexander, S.Y., Selwood, T.S. and Cross, G.F. (1995) Use of polymerase chain reaction for the detection of *Chlamydia trachomatis* in clinical specimens and its comparison to commercially available tests. *Genitourinary Medicine*, **71**(3), 169–71.

Matthews, R.S., Pandit, P.G., Bonigal, S.D., Wise, R., and Radcliffe, K.W. (1993) Evaluation of an enzyme-linked immunoassay and confirmatory test for the detection of *Chlamydia trachomatis* in male urine samples. *Genitourinary Medicine*, **69** (1), 47–50.

Moller, B.R., Herrmann, B., Ibsen, H.H.W. *et al.* (1990) Occurrence of *Ureaplasma urealyticus* and *Mycoplasma hominis* in non-gonococcal urethritis before and after treatment in a double blind trial of ofloxacin vs erythromycin. *Scandinavian Journal of Infectious Diseases*, **22/68**(Supp.), 31–4.

Murray, P.R., Drew, W.L., Kobayashi, G.S. and Thompson, J.H. (1990) *Medical Microbiology*, Wolfe, USA.

Nilsen, A., Halsos, A., Johansen, A. *et al.* (1992) A double blind study of single dose azithromycin and doxycycline in the treatment of chlamydial urethritis in males. *Genitourinary Medicine*, **68**(5), 325–7.

Radcliffe, K.W., Rowen, D., Mercey, D.E. *et al.* (1990) Is a test of cure necessary following treatment for cervical infection with *Chlamydia trachomatis*? *Genitourinary Medicine*, **66**(6), 444–6.

Rahm, V.A., Odlind, V. and Pettersson, R. (1991) *Chlamydia trachomatis* in sexually active teenage girls. Factors related to genital chlamydial infection: a prospective study. *Genitourinary Medicine*, **67**(4), 317–21.

Svensson, O.-L., Mares, I. and Olsson, S.-E. (1991) Detection of *Chlamydia trachomatis* in urinary samples from women. *Genitourinary Medicine*, **67**(2), 117–19.

Szarewski, A., Pompey, A., Bertrand, J. and Bradbeer, C. (1989) Use of the cytobrush for concurrent endocervical cytology and chlamydia sampling. *Genitourinary Medicine*, **66**(3), 205–7.

Whatley, J.D., Thin, R.N., Mumtaz, G. and Ridgway, G.L. (1991) Azithromycin vs doxycycline in the treatment of non-gonococcal urethritis. *International Journal of STD and AIDS*, **2**(4), 248–51.

White, D.J., Mann, C.H., Matthews, R.S. *et al.* (1993) The value of tests of cure following cervical chlamydia infection. *International Journal of STD and AIDS*, **4**(1), 5–7.

WHO (1989) Sexually transmitted disease treatment strategies. W.H.O. consultation on the development of sexually transmitted disease treatment strategies. WHO/VDT 98.447.

Young, H., Moyes, A., Lough, H. *et al.* (1991) Preliminary evaluation of 'Clearview Chlamydia' for the rapid detection of chlamydial antigen in cervical secretions. *Genitourinary Medicine*, **67**(2), 120–3.

9	# Non-specific urethritis

OBJECTIVES

1. To list the main microbiological causes of non-specific urethritis (NSU).
2. To describe the modes of transmission of the microorganisms associated with NSU.
3. To recognize the usual signs and symptoms of NSU.
4. To state the main methods of detection of NSU and the organisms associated with this condition.
5. To describe the common treatment regimes for NSU.
6. To explain the causes of persistence and recurrence of NSU.
7. To understand the importance of follow-up with this condition.

SUMMARY

Non-specific urethritis is also sometimes known as 'non-gonococcal urethritis', meaning urethritis caused by an organism other than *Neisseria gonorrhoeae*. Some authors treat these two conditions as separate entities but here they will be considered as one, because the causes, diagnosis and treatments are identical.

Non-specific urethritis is the second most common condition in men seen in GUM clinics in England. It can be caused by infectious and non-infectious agents.

Several microorganisms and their routes of transmission are discussed in this chapter:

- *Chlamydia trachomatis* (mentioned here but discussed more fully in Chapter 8)
- *Ureaplasma urealyticum*
- *Mycoplasma hominis*

- *Trichomonas vaginalis*
- miscellaneous microorganisms

The symptomology, diagnosis and treatment regimes of NSU are also discussed.

EPIDEMIOLOGY

The incidence of NSU in England is in decline at present (Department of Health, 1995). Data are only available for the five years from 1989 to 1994 but they show that the number of new cases in this period has dropped from 77,260 to 65,974. These figures also include epidemiological treatment of NSU, which must be taken into account when analysing the data.

As previously discussed, *Chlamydia trachomatis* is one of the main causes of NSU. It is believed that this microorganism is responsible for 25–58% cases of NSU. Other detectable organisms are responsible for another 5% of cases and in the remainder of cases the cause is unknown.

In England the incidence of epididymitis, a possible complication of NSU, has remained steady since 1989. In 1994, 118 of 1,524 new cases of epididymitis were found to be caused by *Chlamydia trachomatis* and 23 cases by *Neisseria gonorrhoeae*. In 17 cases both these organisms were found to be present. The remaining 1,366 cases were of non-specific cause. There may be a degree of underdiagnosing of *Chlamydia trachomatis*, as men are not always routinely tested for this.

Certain demographic trends have been observed (Csonka, 1990):

- NSU appears to be more common in Caucasians.
- Peak incidence is in the age group 20–24.
- Men with NSU are more often married and of a higher socioeconomic group.
- NSU is more common in men who have had it before.

MICROBIOLOGY

Chlamydia trachomatis appears to be the leading cause of NSU. The microbiology of this organism is dealt with in Chapter 8. In this chapter the focus is on the other known or possible causes of NSU.

Ureaplasma urealyticum

This is one of the smallest free-living bacteria and belongs to the family Mycoplasmataceae. It has no cell wall, which makes it resistant to penicillins, cephalosporins and other antibiotics that affect the cell wall. This organism replicates by binary fission. Although there are over 14 serotypes of the organism it is thought that only one causes urethritis, serotype 4. It is thought that this organism is responsible for 10% of NSU cases.

The incidence of this organism increases after puberty, corresponding to sexual activity. About 45% of men and 75% of women are colonized with the organism, making diagnosis difficult (Murray *et al.*, 1990).

Mycoplasma hominis

This organism also belongs to the family Mycoplasmataceae and has similar characteristics to ureaplasmas. Although thought to play a part in NSU, *Mycoplasma hominis* appears to be part of the normal flora of the urethra. Fifteen per cent of men and women are colonized with this organism (Murray *et al.*, 1990).

Other anaerobic bacteria

Bacteroides ureolyticus was once suspected to be a cause of NSU. However, it has been observed that this organism is a commensal in the male urethra (Woolley *et al.*, 1990a). Some of the bacteria causing anaerobic vaginosis have also been implicated in NSU but this link is far from proven (Woolley *et al.*, 1990a).

Trichomonas vaginalis

This has been found to be the cause of NSU in a few cases. This organism is difficult to isolate from the male urethra and often can be implicated only if there is a rapid response to treatment with metronidazole.

Miscellaneous microorganisms

All the following microorganisms have at some time been implicated as causes of NSU but their role remains unproven:

- *Corynebacterium genitalium*
- *Haemophilus parainfluenzae*
- *Candida*
- *Herpes simplex*
- Meningococcus
- *Bacteroides species*
- Group B haemolytic streptococcus (the main concern with this group being the potential to cause neonatal infection)
- organisms that cause urinary tract infections

It is important to recognize that there may be non-infective causes of NSU, as follows.

Penile trauma

This can occur during sex or by squeezing and close inspection of the meatus. Sometimes following an episode of NSU, men inspect the penis for discharge without realising that this manipulation itself may cause damage to the lining of the urethra and hence subsequent symptoms of NSU.

Allergies

Some men display allergic reactions to condoms or spermicidal preparations, resulting in symptoms of NSU.

Foreign bodies

Foreign bodies lodged in the urethra are a well recognized phenomenon among men attending GUM clinics. Objects range from wire and safety pins to matchsticks and pencils. It is dangerous to insert any foreign body into the urethra as the delicate lining will be damaged, leaving it susceptible to secondary infection. Symptoms similar to NSU will be experienced; however, if the object is some way into the urethra, diagnosis may be difficult. This is further hampered by the individual's embarrassment and reluctance to disclose the true nature of the problem.

Rings

Rings or other jewellery in the genitals have the potential to cause inflammation and secondary infection. 'Prince Albert' rings in particular, which are inserted through the urethra, may cause symptoms of NSU.

TRANSMISSION

Sexual intercourse is the route of transmission for most of the causative organisms of NSU although the path of infection seems more complex than that of gonorrhoea. It has been suggested that host factors may be important in sensitizing the male urethra to microorganisms present in the female genital tract. Many of these organisms may be harmless commensals until there is a shift in the health status of the individual, at which point these organisms can become pathogenic.

NSU appears to be much less common in gay men, with gonorrhoea more often the cause of urethral symptoms among this group.

It is known that orogenital contact can also transmit genital pathogens such as gonorrhoea and can lead to the development of NSU. In addition Meningococcus, Group B haemolytic streptococcus and other bacteria (for example, *Streptococcus mitis*) can be transmitted in that way (McGowan *et al.*, 1991).

SIGNS AND SYMPTOMS

The incubation period of NSU varies according to the causative organism and therefore is often difficult to ascertain. It is reported to range from a few days to six weeks but is usually 2–3 weeks.

The main symptoms of NSU are:

● urethral discharge
● variable degrees of pyuria
● dysuria

If left untreated or the man is initially asymptomatic, the following complications can arise.

Acute epididymitis

This usually manifests as unilateral swelling and pain in the epididymis. *Chlamydia trachomatis* and *Neisseria gonorrhoeae* are the most common known causes of epididymitis. However, no causative organism has been identified for the majority of cases. *Mycoplasma hominis* and ureaplasmas have also been suggested as possible causes.

Prostatitis

At present there is little conclusive evidence to suggest that either *Mycoplasma hominis* or ureaplasmas are the cause of some prostatitis. Acute bacterial prostatitis can be characterized by:

● sudden chills
● pyrexia
● malaise
● symptoms of bladder outlet obstruction
● urinary frequency
● occasionally urinary retention

Chronic bacterial prostatitis may present with vaguer symptoms and disturbances of bladder function such as:

● frequent and urgent micturition
● intermittent dysuria

- post-micturition dribbling
- post-ejaculatory pain
- haematospermia
- reactive arthropathy (usually associated with chlamydia infection)

DIAGNOSIS

In a GUM clinic several methods may be used to detect NSU. It is helpful for men to have held their urine for at least two hours before attending the clinic. This allows build-up of secretions and therefore increases the likelihood of accurate diagnosis. It may be advised that specimens should be taken in the morning prior to micturition in order to maximize the chance of detecting polymorphonuclear leucocytes (Terry *et al.*, 1991). This indication of inflammation suggests the presence of an infection but further testing is necessary to establish the exact microbiological cause.

The main methods of diagnosis are:

Gram stained slide

A sample of discharge from the urethra is obtained with a plastic loop and smeared on to a microscope slide. This is then Gram stained and microscopically examined under high power ($\times 1000$). A diagnosis of NSU can be made if there are more than four polymorphonuclear leucocytes in more than five fields. This method has been shown to be a sensitive and specific indicator of NSU (Terry *et al.*, 1991).

It is important to carefully prepare and systematically examine the slide in order to eliminate observer variation as far as possible and to detect any other microorganisms, e.g. gonococcus.

Two-glass urine test

Urine is passed into two glasses. Any specks or threads in the first glass may indicate an anterior urethritis. Specks or threads in the second glass may indicate a problem in the posterior urethra.

Testing for chlamydia

A urethral specimen is obtained and sent to the laboratory for chlamydia testing.

Testing for gonorrhoea

It is very important that the Gram stained specimen is also examined for the presence of *Neisseria gonorrhoeae* and a culture sent to the laboratory.

If this is omitted, an incorrect diagnosis may result and inappropriate treatment be administered. After the treatment of gonorrhoea, symptoms may persist; this is known as post-gonococcal urethritis (PGU) and is an indication of concurrent NSU, for which appropriate treatment is required.

It is difficult to isolate other microorganisms associated with NSU, such as *Ureaplasma urealyticum* and *Mycoplasma hominis* and many laboratories do not investigate these microorganisms. Moreover the cost and effectiveness of the treatment of NSU negates the benefit of culturing these organisms.

TREATMENT

Erythromycin and tetracyclines have long been the drugs of choice for the treatment of NSU (Higgins, 1993). Many regimes incorporating these drugs are used, commonly:

- oxytetracycline 500 mg 2–4 times a day for seven days
- triple tetracycline 300 mg twice daily
- doxycycline 100 mg twice daily for seven days
  or 200 mg stat, then 100 mg once daily for nine days
- erythromycin 500 mg 2–4 times a day

The lower dosages are adequate and may increase compliance. Even though oxytetracycline may be the cheapest, an alternative that is taken twice daily may be preferred to improve compliance.

Recent work has demonstrated that azithromycin can be used in the treatment of NSU in a single dose of 1 g or 500 mg loading dose followed by 250 mg daily for two days. The response was better for the three-day regime (95%) than for the single dose (76%) (Whatley *et al.*, 1991). This method of treatment offers advantages in patient compliance.

In regard to drug resistance, some tetracycline-resistant ureaplasmas have been identified but they would not account for all persistent NSU.

With the role of anaerobic bacteria still unclear, there is little evidence to suggest that treatment with metronidazole will reduce the number of cases of persistent urethritis or the relapse of patients with NSU (Woolley *et al.*, 1990b).

Some important considerations in the treatment of NSU are as follows:

- NSU caused by chlamydia responds better to treatment than does NSU caused by other organisms.
- If sexual activity occurs while the patient is taking medication and symptoms persist, it is difficult to distinguish between reinfection and relapse.

- A complete cure is not certain even after eradication of chlamydia and ureaplasmas. Unidentified microorganisms may be the cause.
- Some sites may be protected from treatment, e.g. the prostate gland.
- In cases of NSU with non-infective causes, such as penile trauma due to squeezing and inspection of the penis or high alcohol consumption, antibiotic treatment will not provide a cure.
- Psychological factors must be considered, especially in men with persistent symptoms.
- There is some evidence that it may be possible for *Chlamydia trachomatis* to remain latent inside the host cells.
- In some cases symptoms may resolve spontaneously.

Recent work has shown that a significant number of men with NSU treat themselves with their own or others' stored medication before presenting to a GUM clinic (Carlin and Barton, 1995). This makes accurate diagnosis, treatment and contact tracing difficult and increases the likelihood of adverse reactions if individuals take medication not prescribed for themselves.

It is recognized that sexual partners of men with NSU should be treated epidemiologically and that female partners of men with NSU should be screened for chlamydia and treated simultaneously. There is some evidence that treatment of women whose partners have non-chlamydial NSU prevents recurrence in the male partners. This suggests that other microorganisms can be harboured and transmitted by female partners.

It is well recognized that NSU is not always easily curable. Persistence and recurrence may well be part of its natural history and are not necessarily determined by a microbiological cause.

FOLLOW-UP

Follow-up is an essential part of the treatment process for NSU. A follow-up visit is usually advised one week after finishing the course of treatment. On this visit it is usually the nurse's responsibility to check the following:

- Compliance with treatment. This requires good communication skills as people may be embarrassed or anxious if they have failed to comply with treatment. Explanations of the consequences of untreated infections are required. Treatment regimes can appear confusing and complicated to those unfamiliar with them.
- Resolution of symptoms.
- Results of the tests carried out on the first visit will be available and treatment can be changed if necessary. Further treatment may not

always be necessary; for example, if chlamydia is detected, NSU treatment should have been sufficient. If any other organisms are detected, such as gonorrhoea, further treatment will be needed. If a diagnosis of a definite sexually transmitted infection is made, further advice and counselling is important. A diagnosis of NSU could possibly be attributed to a non-infective or non-sexually transmitted cause in some cases.

- Contact tracing. Partners need to be examined and treated to reduce the pool of infection and to prevent pelvic inflammatory disease (see Chapter 10). Sometimes advice is needed on ways to tell partners that they need to attend the clinic. The importance of contact tracing must be emphasized.
- A Gram stained slide is checked for the presence of polymorphonuclear leucocytes.
- A two-glass urine test is performed.

Information about safer sexual practices, including the recommending of condoms, is important in preventing further episodes of NSU and other infections.

GLOSSARY

Arthropathy	Any disease of a joint
Epididymitis	Inflammation of the epididymus
Haematospermia	Blood in the seminal fluid
Prostatitis	Inflammation of the prostate gland
Pyuria	The presence of neutrophils (pus) in the urine
Serotype	A subgroup of a genus of microorganisms identifiable by their surface antigens
Urethritis	Inflammation of the urethra

REFERENCES

Carlin, E.M. and Barton, S.E. (1995) How common is self-treatment in non-gonococcal urethritis? *Genitourinary Medicine*, **71**(6), 400–1.

Csonka, G.W. (1990) 'Non-specific' genital infection, in *Sexually Transmitted Diseases – A Textbook of Genitourinary Medicine* (eds G.W. Csonka and J.K. Oates), Baillière Tindall, London.

Department of Health (1995) *Statistical Bulletin: Sexually Transmitted Diseases, England 1994*. Bulletin 1995/16.

Higgins, S. (1993) Diagnosis and management of non-gonococcal urethritis. *British Journal of Sexual Medicine.* **20**(4), 16–21.

McGowan, I., Radcliffe, K.W., Bingham, J.S. *et al.* (1991) Non-gonococcal urethritis in men practising 'safe sex'. *Genitourinary Medicine*, **67**(1), 70–1.

Murray, P.R., Drew, W.L., Kobayashi, G.S. and Thompson, J.H. (1990) *Medical Microbiology*, Wolfe, USA.

Terry, P.M., Holland, S., Olden, D. and O'Connell, S. (1991) Diagnosing non-gonococcal urethritis: the Gram-stained urethral smear in perspective. *International Journal of STD and AIDS*, **2**(4), 272–5.

Whatley, J.D., Thin, R.N., Mumtaz, G. and Ridgway, G.L. (1991) Azithromycin vs doxycycline in the treatment of non-gonococcal urethritis. *International Journal of STD and AIDS*, **2**(4), 248–51.

Woolley, P.D., Kinghorn, G.R., Talbot, M.D. and Duerden, B.I. (1990a) Microbiological flora in men with non-gonococcal urethritis with particular reference to anaerobic bacteria. *International Journal of STD and AIDS*, **1**(2), 122–5.

Woolley, P.D., Kinghorn, G.R., Talbot, M.D. and Duerden, B.I. (1990b) Efficacy of combined metronidazole and triple tetracycline therapy in the treatment of non-gonococcal urethritis. *International Journal of STD and AIDS*, **1**(1), 35–7.

OBJECTIVES

1. To recognize the main microbiological causes of pelvic inflammatory disease (PID).
2. To explain the modes of transmission of organisms associated with PID.
3. To describe the main signs, symptoms and stages of PID.
4. To list the methods of diagnosis of PID.
5. To identify the main complications and implications of this condition.
6. To describe the common treatment regimes for PID.
7. To recognize the importance of follow-up for patients with PID and for their partners.

SUMMARY

Pelvic inflammatory disease can be described as inflammation of the upper genital tract. It includes several inflammatory conditions including salpingitis, salpingo-oophoritis and endometritis and is usually bilateral. The distinction between these conditions is not often made and 'pelvic inflammatory disease' is used as a general term encompassing all of these.

Pelvic inflammatory disease is difficult to diagnose as many women have vague and mild symptoms. It is important to take all symptoms seriously, however, as even women who are asymptomatic or who experience only mild symptoms may still face severely damaged uterine tubes and impaired fertility.

EPIDEMIOLOGY

It is reported that the incidence of pelvic infection in the United Kingdom is on the increase (Department of Health, 1995). Data relating to pelvic infection has been officially collected only since 1989 so a longer-term view is not possible. However, in England the number of new cases seen in GUM clinics rose from 4,954 in 1989 to 7,690 in 1994.

In England in 1994, 575 reported cases of pelvic infection were caused by *Chlamydia trachomatis*, confirming this as the most common known cause of PID. In the same year 89 new cases of PID were caused by *Neisseiria gonorrhoeae*. In addition 77 new cases of PID were caused by infection with both these organisms and 6,949 cases had a non-specific cause.

It must be noted that there may be a high degree of underreporting of both PID and other conditions seen in GUM clinics. Many women attending GP surgeries and family planning clinics with pelvic symptoms may be treated with antibiotics but the condition never officially diagnosed or reported. In addition some women may not seek any medical opinion at all, believing the symptoms to be a normal part of the menstrual cycle.

MICROBIOLOGY

Chlamydia trachomatis

Pelvic inflammatory disease is a complication of untreated *Chlamydia trachomatis* infection. The long-term consequences of this could be recurrent pain, ectopic pregnancy and impaired fertility. This organism is recognized as one of the most common known causes of PID. See Chapter 8 for more detail on *Chlamydia trachomatis*.

It has been noted that PID caused by chlamydia may run a clinically less severe course than other forms of PID, e.g. those caused *by Neisseiria gonorrhoeae*. However, even episodes of chlamydial PID which have been asymptomatic can have serious consequences such as tubal obstruction and impaired fertility (Patton *et al.*, 1989). In addition this 'silent' PID may predispose the woman to ectopic pregnancy (Walters *et al.*, 1988).

Neisseria gonorrhoeae

Before the availability of antibiotics there was some evidence that PID caused by gonorrhoea was self-limiting, running a course of 10–14 days before resolving to leave damaged uterine tubes. It is suggested that a toxin released by the gonococci disables the cilia lining the uterine tubes, leaving them open to infection by other secondary organisms (MacLean, 1995).

The signs and symptoms of gonococcal PID are more pronounced. However, it has proved difficult to isolate the organism in many cases, perhaps because of its self-limiting characteristics. See Chapter 7 for more details on gonorrhoea.

Mycoplasmas and ureaplasmas

Although these organisms have been isolated from the uterine tubes in cases of PID, their role is unclear.

Haemophilus influenzae

Again the role of this organism is unclear but it has been suggested that the route of transmission may be orogenital sex (Paavonen *et al.*, 1986). *Mycoplasma pneumoniae* and Group A streptococci have also been isolated from uterine tubes and are believed to be transmitted the same way.

Endogenous aerobic and anaerobic bacteria

Anaerobes such as *Bacteroides fragilis* and peptococci are the most common. The main aerobes are *Escherichia coli* and streptococci. It appears that many of these bacteria are secondary invaders. However, a link between bacterial vaginosis and PID has been suggested, especially in women whose uterine tubes have been previously affected by chlamydia or gonorrhoea (Eschenbach *et al.*, 1988).

Actinomyces spp.

The role of this Gram-positive bacterium in PID is unclear. For women not using intrauterine contraceptive devices it appears to be of little significance. For those using these devices there may be a small risk of PID and abscess formation if this organism is present. In these cases treatment may be given to eradicate the organism, usually penicillin, tetracycline or erythromycin, and the intrauterine device removed.

Mycobacterium tuberculosis

This is rare in developed countries and half of the women affected have a focus of infection elsewhere. It is treated with anti-tubercular therapy and can result in ectopic pregnancy.

Herpes simplex

Rarely this may be the cause of PID.

TRANSMISSION

The cervix in its usual state provides a good barrier against infection travelling into the uterus. In certain situations this barrier is breached in some way, allowing entry of microorganisms:

- Childbirth or miscarriage leaves the cervix open and possibly damaged.
- Surgical instrumentation of the uterus, for example in termination of pregnancy.
- Intrauterine contraceptive devices.
- Previous attacks of PID seem to reduce resistance, with the subsequent episode often due to normal vaginal or bowel flora.
- During sexual intercourse, microorganisms may be propelled through the cervix by a microbial vector, e.g. *Trichomonas vaginalis*, or sucked into the cervix by pressure changes during sex. More likely, however, is the transport of microorganisms by spermatazoa into the upper genital tract.

The initial cause and progression of PID can appear confusing. To clarify this, Hare (1990) describes 3 types of PID:

1. Primary PID:

   - This ccurs in the undamaged pelvis of usually a younger woman.
   - Microorganisms use a transport mechanism to penetrate the cervix.
   - Infection is commonly caused by sexually transmitted agents.

2. Secondary PID:

   - The cervical barrier has been compromised in some other way, e.g. by instrumentation or childbirth.
   - The infection is more likely due to aerobic and anaerobic vaginal and bowel flora.

3. Recurrent PID:

   - Previous infection means an increased risk of recurrent infection.

SIGNS AND SYMPTOMS

The symptoms of PID are varied and differ in severity. The main recognized symptoms are:

- mucopurulent vaginal discharge
- abdominal pain
- dyspareunia
- bleeding during intercourse
- lower back pain
- tenderness in the lower abdomen
- fever
- urinary disturbance
- vomiting

On examination there may be:

- tenderness on bimanual examination
- abdominal mass
- vaginal discharge

If the condition is left untreated, certain short-term and long-term complications may arise.

Short-term complications

Fitz-Hugh-Curtis syndrome

This occurs in about 5% of cases of PID and takes the form of a peri-hepatitis, usually chlamydial or gonococcal in origin. On laparoscopy, oedema of the liver capsule and adhesions to the peritoneum are evident.

Pelvic abscess

This occurs in up to one-third of all cases of PID and is detected by the palpation of an adnexal mass, confirmed by ultrasound or laparoscopy. Antibiotics may reduce this but surgical intervention may be necessary to remove it.

Long-term complications

Chronic pain

Often the exact origin of this pain is difficult to ascertain. It may be due to recurrence of infection or adhesions and scarring in the pelvic cavity. This may cause pain on intercourse or at times during the menstrual cycle when the pelvic organs move in response to hormonal influence.

Recurrence

After one episode of PID, subsequent attacks are more likely.

Ectopic pregnancy

Due to damage to the uterine tubes, ectopic pregnancy is more likely in women who have had previous episodes of PID.

Impaired fertility

The likelihood of impaired fertility increases after each attack of PID.

DIAGNOSIS

The diagnosis of PID is difficult due to the often vague symptoms, and the spontaneous resolution in some cases (Stacey and Munday, 1994). Laboratory investigations are necessary to attempt to identify the causative agent of PID. In GUM clinics the first line of investigation is the taking of endocervical swabs as part of a full screen for sexually transmitted infections. In the case of suspected PID, gonorrhoea and chlamydia swabs are of particular importance. If the woman is hospitalized, other investigations are:

- blood cultures
- specimens from the uterine tubes on laparoscopy
- specimens from the endometrial cavity
- peritoneal fluid from the rectovaginal pouch

In practice the last two investigations are rarely carried out.

It is recognized that the clinical diagnosis of lower abdominal pain in women is difficult; however, combinations of the signs and symptoms listed above improve the accuracy of diagnosis.

Hager and colleagues (1983) suggested the following clinical criteria for the diagnosis and grading of PID. A diagnosis of salpingitis requires all of the following:

1. Abdominal tenderness on palpation, with or without rebound.
2. Excitation tenderness on moving the cervix and uterus.
3. Adnexal tenderness on bimanual palpation.

— plus one more of the following:

4. Gram stain of the endocervix positive for gonorrhoea.
5. Pyrexia greater than 38°C.
6. Leucocytosis greater than 10,000 WBC/mm^3.
7. Purulent fluid (containing WBC) from the peritoneal cavity, usually obtained by laparoscopy.
8. Pelvic abscess or inflammatory complex detected by bimanual examination or by ultrasound.

Clinical examination will suggest one of the following stages:

I. Uncomplicated (limited to tubes and/or ovaries), with or without pelvic peritonitis.
II. Complicated (inflammatory mass or tubal or tubo-ovarian abscess).
III. Spread to structures beyond the pelvis, e.g. ruptured tubo-ovarian abscess.

Routine laparoscopy may overcome many diagnostic problems. However, to use this surgical procedure on all women with suspected PID is impractical, and unacceptable to many women. It is rarely performed on women with mild symptoms of PID which resolve after treatment with antibiotics.

In some cases, however, laparoscopy is indicated:

- if the woman is severely ill
- in women with recurrent symptoms
- in older women when endometriosis and malignancy are likely
- where ectopic pregnancy is suspected
- in women claiming to have had no sexual intercourse

One interesting diagnostic marker is that the erythrocyte sedimentation rate (ESR) is markedly elevated in chlamydial PID compared to other forms.

TREATMENT

Antimicrobial therapy is obviously the preferred choice; however, this must be started quickly, often before the microbiological results are available. This means that the antibiotics prescribed must be broad spectrum to cover the majority of organisms.

A useful theoretical guide to antibiotic regimes was devised by Bell and James (1980):

(I)   Maximum theoretical cover (97%): three antibiotics.
(II)   96% cover with two parenteral antibiotics.
(III) 94% cover with two oral antibiotics.
(IV) 84% cover with one parenteral antibiotic.
(V)   74% cover with one oral antibiotic.

Ciprofloxacin along with doxycycline and metronidazole is a regime currently used for the treatment of PID. Ciprofloxacin will treat gonorrhoea and other significant organisms such as streptococci; however, its action against anaerobic bacteria is limited. Doxycycline is a broad spectrum antibiotic and is used for its action against chlamydia and mycoplasmas. Metronidazole is added due to its action against anaerobic organisms such as *Bacteroides fragilis* and *Trichomonas vaginalis*. This regime will ensure antibiotic cover for most of the causative organisms of PID.

A suggested treatment regime for complicated PID is (Heinonen *et al.*, 1989):

- ciprofloxacin 200 mg 12 hourly, (IV) for two days followed by 750 mg orally for 14 days;
- doxycycline 100 mg 12 hourly, (IV) for two days followed by oral therapy for 14 days;

- metronidazole 500 mg 12 hourly, (IV) for two days followed by oral therapy for 14 days.

Often in GUM clinics, uncomplicated PID is treated with a less rigorous regime of antibiotics. A suitable combination may be:

- ampicillin 3 g
- probenecid 1 g
- doxycycline 100 mg twice daily for 10–14 days
- metronidazole 400 mg three times daily for ten days

FOLLOW-UP

For both uncomplicated and complicated PID, follow-up is important in order to monitor the effectiveness of treatment. Unfortunately, damage to the uterine tubes is irreversible and often results in impaired fertility. In view of this it is vital that the mode of transmission of the organisms causing this disease is understood so as to prevent reinfection. The serious consequences of untreated or recurrent PID must be explained to women and their sexual partners, and promotion of safer sex is vital.

Contact tracing is essential to prevent reinfection; unfortunately this is often neglected in other health care settings. The investigation and treatment of sexual partners is sometimes omitted, particularly when patients are hospitalized. This highlights a need for departments of gynaecology and GUM clinics to liaise to prevent reinfection and to provide a consistent approach to the management of this complex condition. This is an opportunity for nurses to forge and maintain links with other disciplines and to share their specialist knowledge with others. Joint working practices between departments improve the quality of care and allow nurses to broaden their knowledge of other specialist areas.

In addition to patient education, the education of other health care professionals should be encouraged, e.g. general practitioners and family planning nurses and doctors. The importance of referral must be emphasized in these settings. If pelvic infection or any other sexually transmitted infection is suspected, referral to a GUM clinic is preferred, so that extensive tests and investigations can be carried out. This will enable prompt diagnosis and commencement of treatment and limit the possibility of permanent damage.

In many GUM clinics a formal or informal nurse triage system operates whereby individuals arriving without appointments can be assessed by an experienced member of the nursing staff almost immediately. If pelvic infection is suspected by the nurse the individual will be seen by the doctor the same day. Referring agents must be encouraged to use this service rather than risk misdiagnosis and delayed or inappropriate treatment for a suspected pelvic infection.

GLOSSARY

Adhesion	Union between two surfaces normally separate, usually the result of inflammation when fibrous tissue forms
Adnexa	Adjoining parts of the body
Dyspareunia	Painful sexual intercourse for women
Ectopic pregnancy	The fertilized egg becomes implanted in an abnormal site, such as the uterine tube, pelvis or abdomen, instead of in the uterus
Endometritis	Inflammation of the endometrium
Laparoscopy	Viewing of the abdominal cavity by passing an endoscope through the abdominal wall
Leucocytosis	An abnormally high number of leucocytes in the blood, often a response to infection
Palpation	The examination of organs by touch or pressure of the hand over the part in question
Pyosalpinx	The presence of pus in the uterine tube
Rebound tenderness	A clinical sign of inflammation. Gentle but increasing pressure is applied to the abdomen then suddenly released. A definite pain felt in another part of the abdomen suggests disease.
Salpingo-oophoritis	Inflammation of the uterine tubes and ovaries

REFERENCES

Bell, T.A. and James, J.F. (1980) Computer assisted analysis of the therapy of acute salpingitis. *American Journal of Obstetrics and Gynaecology*, **138**, 1048–54.

Department of Health (1995) *Statistical Bulletin: Sexually Transmitted Diseases, England 1994.* Bulletin 1995/16.

Eschenbach, D.A., Hillier S., Critchlow C. *et al.* (1988) Diagnosis and clinical management of bacterial vaginosis. *American Journal of Obstetrics and Gynaecology*, **158**, 819–28.

Hager, W.D., Eschenbach, D.A., Spence, M.R. and Sweet, R.L. (1983) Criteria for diagnosis and grading of salpingitis. *Obstetrics and Gynaecology*, **158**, 819–28.

Hare, J. (1990) Pelvic inflammatory disease, in *Sexually Transmitted Diseases: A Textbook of Genitourinary Medicine* (eds G.W. Csonka and J.K. Oates), Baillière Tindall, London.

Heinonen, P.K., Teisala, K., Miettinen, A. *et al.* (1989) A comparison of ciprofloxacin with doxycycline plus metronidazole in the treatment of acute pelvic inflammatory disease. *Scandinavian Journal of Infectious Diseases*, **60**, 66–73.

MacLean, A. (1995) Pelvic infection, in *Dewhurst's Textbook of Obstetrics and Gynaecology for Postgraduates*, 5th edn (ed. C. Whitfield), Blackwell Science, Oxford.

Paavonen, J., Lehtinen, M., Teisala, K. *et al.* (1986) *Haemophilus influenzae* causes purulent salpingitis. *American Journal of Obstetrics and Gynaecology*, **151**, 338–9.

Patton, D.L., Moore, D.E., Spadoni, L.R. *et al.* (1989) A comparison of the Fallopian tubes' response to overt and silent salpingitis. *Obstetrics and Gynaecology*, **73**, 622–30.

Stacey, C.M. and Munday, P.E. (1994) Abdominal pain in women attending a genitourinary medicine clinic: who has PID? *International Journal of STD and AIDS*, **5**(5), 338–42.

Walters, M.D., Eddy, C.A., Gibbs, R.S. *et al.* (1988) Antibodies to *C. trachomatis* and risk from tubal pregnancy. *American Journal of Obstetrics and Gynaecology*, **159**, 942–6.

OBJECTIVES

1. To explain the aetiology of genital warts.
2. To describe the mode of transmission of the human papillomavirus (HPV).
3. To recognize the different types of warts and other signs and symptoms associated with them.
4. To explain the diagnosis and methods of detection of genital warts and HPV.
5. To describe the common treatment regimes for genital warts.
6. To recognize the complications of HPV, particularly in relation to its effect on the cervix.
7. To explain the importance of follow-up for clients with genital warts.

SUMMARY

Genital warts are otherwise known as 'condyloma acuminata'. They are one of the most common conditions of both men and women seen in GUM clinics.This chapter describes the aetiology of HPV, its transmission and its manifestations. Complications of infection with this virus are discussed, with particular reference to its effect on the female cervix. Methods of detection of the virus and treatment options and regimes are described, and the importance of follow-up is discussed.

EPIDEMIOLOGY

It is reported that the number of cases of wart virus infection has steadily increased in England over the last decade (Department of Health, 1995).

In fact the figure of 86,725 cases in 1994 is almost double the figure of 44,050 cases in 1984. From 1989 first attacks of wart virus infection were reported separately from recurrences. These yearly totals have remained constant at around 43% of total genital wart cases. Similar numbers of cases were reported for men and women.

In 1994 it appears that the majority of the cases (71%) of first-attack wart virus infection occurred in the 20–34 age group, although 16.5%, occurred in the 16 and under group. This has implications for the sex education of young people.

It must be emphasized that these figures represent only the reported cases of wart virus infection. Cases diagnosed at other centres, such as GP surgeries and family planning clinics, may not be reported. Moreover, many people may not know that they have wart virus infection because they have no visible signs of warts; therefore, these cases also will go unreported.

MICROBIOLOGY

Genital warts were first described in Roman times; even then they were suspected to be sexually transmitted. The ancient Greeks named them 'condylomata acuminata' because of their shape: 'condylomata' means 'rounded' and 'acuminata' means 'pointed'.

Genital warts are caused by the human papillomaviruses, members of the larger papovirus group. These viruses are icosahedral in shape, do not have an envelope and are approximately 50 nm in size. They contain a circular double strand of DNA, and it is from this DNA that the papillomaviruses are typed, as the viruses cannot be grown in cell culture. To date, at least 50 types of HPV have been identified in this way. The incubation period of HPV is difficult to ascertain but is estimated to range between three weeks and eight months. The route of transmission is difficult to establish in some cases due to this variable incubation period. In some cases the virus may remain latent for many years.

Papillomaviruses infect mucosal epithelium and replicate causing excessive growth of the epithelial cells, which results in the familiar manifestation of warts. Some papillomaviruses may be involved in both benign and malignant tumour growth.

Ninety per cent of genital warts are caused by HPV types 6 and 11 but it is known that HPV types 16 and 18 are also sexually transmitted and are linked with intraepithelial cervical neoplasia and cervical cancer. Up to 70% of mild abnormalities caused by these types return to normal but the disease can progress to severe abnormalities or neoplastic change after 1–4 years. There is much discussion about the role of HPV 16 in the development of cervical cancer. There are three main schools of thought (Gross *et al.*, 1990):

1. HPV 16 plays a highly significant part in the development of anogenital malignancy.
2. HPV 16 causes anogenital malignancy only in the presence of certain co-factors, which are discussed later in this chapter.
3. HPV 16 is of little significance in the development of anogenital malignancy.

It is recognized that immune response is important in the control of HPV. Genital warts proliferate during pregnancy and are more likely to develop in immunosuppressed individuals.

TRANSMISSION

Human papillomavirus is transmitted via sexual intercourse and, it is thought, close genital contact. The virus enters the epithelium usually through a breach in the surface, often caused by trauma, and enters the host cell. Studies have shown that it is unlikely that HPV DNA is transmitted via semen (Nieminen, Koskimies and Paavonen, 1991). Once the virus has entered the epithelial cells it undergoes transformation and proliferates, causing the familiar formation of a wart. The virus is found in the superficial layers of the wart and can infect other epithelial cells when shed. The incubation period of HPV is difficult to determine but may be up to one year.

Using polymerase chain reaction (PCR) methods it has been demonstrated that up to 84% of men can carry HPV on the penis and 80% of women carry HPV on the cervix even if their cervical cytology is apparently normal (Wikstrom *et al.*, 1991). It is thought that the risk of transmission is highest in the first year after the appearance of the warts. Warts in the mouth can be transmitted by oral sex and respiratory tract papillomas can arise by the same transmission route. Both these conditions are rare.

Genital warts have been observed in children. Vulval and perianal warts are more common than penile warts. Often it is difficult to discover the origin of the virus but it may be that the mother had genital warts at the time of delivery. Sexual abuse must also be considered, especially if anogenital warts are present; however, this is not proof of abuse (Oriel, 1988).

A rare disorder, laryngeal papillomatosis, can occur in late infancy, caused by the presence of genital warts in the mother during pregnancy and birth. This condition is significant, for it may become malignant.

SIGNS AND SYMPTOMS

Human papillomavirus can manifest itself in many forms of genital wart. Some descriptions of their appearance are:

- filiform – threadlike
- pedunculated – on a stalk
- sessile – flat and wide based
- flat

Men

The most common sites of genital warts in men are:

- coronal sulcus
- frenum
- prepuce

Other sites are:

- shaft of the penis
- scrotum
- anal and perianal areas
- urethra
- mouth

Anal and perianal warts are often transmitted by anal intercourse, but this is not always the case. As this area of the body is warm and moist, the warts often proliferate and can become quite large. In addition they can spread up into the anal canal where they are more difficult to treat.

Genital warts can also occur in the urethra, where they are known as 'meatal warts'. They can occur here alone or in association with warts elsewhere on the genitals. Often no symptoms are associated with urethral warts but the following have been noted:

- dysuria
- urethral discharge
- urethral bleeding

Other unusual sites are possible:

- Urethral warts do rarely spread up into the bladder.
- Occasionally warts can occur in the mouth, sometimes concurrently with genital warts.
- It has been suggested that HPV can cause a protracted balanitis which does not respond to steroids (Birley *et al.*, 1994). This may be borne in mind as a differential diagnosis of balanoposthitis.

Women

The most common areas for genital warts in women are:

- fourchette
- labia minora
- clitoris
- labia majora
- perianal area
- vagina
- urethra

The cervix can also be affected. In some women HPV can lead to cervical intraepithelial neoplasia (CIN). Cellular changes are detectable on cervical smear testing and may suggest the presence of HPV. In up to two-thirds of cases it would appear that the cells return to normal after a time, but some women develop progressive disease (Handley *et al.*, 1992). It is thought that a different type of wart, a flat wart, is responsible for these changes. These warts may not be visible to the naked eye but can be seen during colposcopy.

The development of cervical squamous cell carcinoma may be due to various co-factors:

- type of HPV
- cigarette smoking
- other cervical infections
- lack of hygiene
- the use of oral contraception
- low vitamin A intake
- number of sexual partners

It is difficult to prove a direct correlation between anogenital warts and cervical squamous cell carcinoma as this may take 15–25 years to develop. Long-term follow-up study of women who have had anogenital warts and cervical pre-neoplasias is needed to clarify this matter.

The appearance of genital warts or proliferation of existing warts during pregnancy is thought to be due to alterations in cell-mediated immune responses.

Complications

Although there are no recognized systemic complications associated with HPV infection, local problems can arise:

- Large warts may ulcerate, become infected or haemorrhage.
- There is a link between mothers having genital warts during pregnancy and their infants having laryngeal papillomas.

- Rarely, giant condylomata occurs, in which the lesion rapidly enlarges the underlying tissue over a wide area.

DIAGNOSIS

Genital warts are usually diagnosed on clinical appearance as there is no convenient, cost-effective screening test available for use in GUM clinics. In both men and women the genital area is examined very carefully for signs of warts. In women a speculum examination is also performed to check the vagina and cervix.

In men meatoscopy can be performed to examine the distal anterior urethra. This is the examination of the anterior urethra using an auroscope. Men with urethral warts almost always have meatal warts; in these cases meatoscopy is recommended for determining the site of the wart's base (Thin, 1992).

Sometimes flat warts may be difficult to distinguish. In this case 5% acetic acid is applied to the area in question. After a few minutes any abnormal areas of skin infected with HPV become white. Wart tissue can also be examined microscopically to reveal the appearance of prickle cells and excess keratin production. Vacuolated squamous epithelial cells may also be present. Under electron microscopy, the papillomavirus itself can be detected. Immunofluorescence and other techniques may be used. It is also possible to detect antibodies to HPV in the blood but in the case of genital warts an inadequate amount of virus is available to use for testing.

As with all sexually transmitted infections it is important to eliminate any other possible infections. A routine screen for sexually transmitted infections is recommended. The presence of inflammatory conditions such as candidiasis may activate the wart virus and decrease the effectiveness of treatment. Therefore it is important to treat such conditions before attempting to treat the warts.

TREATMENT

In many GUM clinics in the United Kingdom the main expertise in wart treatment is found among the nursing staff. Although clients have a medical consultation on their initial visit to the department, the nurses will then take over the treatment of genital warts. On each attendance the progress of the treatment is assessed and modified accordingly. At set intervals a doctor's review will be necessary if the genital warts persist.

It is widely recognized that there is no single most effective method of treatment for genital warts. Individuals respond to different treatments with different degrees of success. Certain factors may affect the response of genital warts to treatment:

1. The number of warts present: if the warts are multiple and widespread they are more difficult to treat.
2. The length of time the warts have been present: warts present for some time have a lower response rate to treatment, usually because the surface of the wart is keratinized, which hinders the absorption of treatment solutions.
3. The site of the warts: Reynolds and colleagues (1993) showed that some clients with genital warts at particular sites had significantly higher failure rates after three months of treatment. These were:

   - women with vaginal warts
   - women with cervical warts
   - men with anal/perineal warts
   - men and women with two or more sites affected

4. In women the hormonal changes of pregnancy can decrease the response to treatment.

Podophyllin

The oldest and most common treatment for genital warts is podophyllin. This resin is extracted from the plants *Podophyllum emodi* and *Podophyllum peltatum*. It is used in a tincture of benzoin compound or as a 10–40% solution in ethanol. Podophyllotoxin is the most active ingredient of podophyllin and this is also available in a pure 0.5% solution as described below.

The mode of action of podophyllin is the interruption of nuclear division, at the metaphase stage of mitosis, in affected cells. The solution is available in strengths of 10% and 25% and is applied directly on to the wart and washed off after four hours. This can be done once or twice a week until the wart has gone. Unfortunately podophyllin has some side effects:

- It can irritate normal skin, so it is important to apply it accurately to affected areas only. The damage to skin can range from local redness to widespread ulceration.
- If large quantities are applied, systemic absorption may occur causing dizziness, abdominal pain, vomiting, diarrhoea and neurological side effects. These effects are rare.
- It may be mutagenic so cannot be used in pregnancy

In addition it is difficult to be sure of the exact concentration of the substance as batches may vary in potency.

Podophyllin must be applied by trained personnel. This means a visit to the GUM clinic once or twice a week. It is widely accepted that if genital warts have not responded to regular applications of podophyllin after an agreed period, alternative treatment should be substituted.

Trichloracetic acid

On application this solution has a coagulation effect, with necrosis of the superficial skin layers. It can be used for small warts but must be applied carefully using a sharpened wooden stick. It burns normal skin, leaving ulceration and scarring. When using this it is advisable to apply Vaseline to the surrounding area to protect the healthy skin.

Podophyllotoxin

This is the active ingredient of podophyllin and is recognized as a treatment for genital warts in a 0.5% solution. Studies have demonstrated that the action of podophyllotoxin is superior to that of podophyllin, showing a quicker clearance of visible genital warts in both men and women (Kinghorn *et al.*, 1993). There are fewer side effects because it is a pure and more stable substance. It may also be used at home, which eliminates the inconvenience of frequent visits to the clinic.

Although the results of studies of podophyllotoxin appear favourable, it is important that individuals treating themselves at home are reviewed by an experienced doctor or nurse to ensure that treatment is applied correctly and that side effects are minimized. In addition this solution is more expensive than podophyllin.

A cream containing 0.5% podophyllotoxin is available for home treatment and has been shown to be as effective as the solution (Sand Petersen *et al.*, 1995). Although the cream is easy to apply, it may cause more adverse reactions as it will be spread over a wider area. Careful monitoring is necessary, as with the solution.

5-Fluorouracil (5-FU)

This chemical is an antimetabolite which prevents normal cell division and is used to treat solid tumours. It can be used to treat intraurethral warts as a 5% cream. It is applied after micturition and at night for 3–8 days. It can cause local soreness.

Cryotherapy

Various forms of cryotherapy are used:

- nitrous oxide
- liquid nitrogen
- carbon dioxide snow

Individual warts are frozen, causing cell destruction. This method is useful for the treatment of large warts. Treatment to the surrounding normal skin should be minimized to prevent soreness. This treatment can be painful both at the time of treatment and afterwards.

Cautery

Local anaesthetic is administered and the warts are cauterized, causing cell destruction. A hyfrecator can also be used, performing electrodessication by high frequency sparking. These treatments must be used with caution so as to minimize scarring.

Surgery

Some genital warts are so extensive that the quickest and most effective method of removal is surgery under general anaesthetic. This is most common for anogenital warts. For preputial warts, circumcision may be recommended.

Carbon dioxide laser

This may be used for warts found on the cervix during colposcopic examination. It requires a local anaesthetic but has a high success rate compared to other therapies. Studies have been conducted using interferons to stimulate cell-mediated immunity, thus reducing the occurrence of genital warts. More work is needed to produce convincing evidence of the effectiveness of such treatments.

Many of the treatments described above can be used in isolation or in combination. It has been noted that in a small number of people genital warts may disappear spontaneously. This may be linked to the presence of HPV specific antibodies and an increase in cell-mediated immunity. However, the mechanisms are not fully understood.

Many male partners of women with anogenital warts never appear to develop lesions themselves. The suggested explanations (Law *et al.*, 1991) are that:

- the men have built up immunity to HPV from past infection;
- the women are no longer infectious.

It is very difficult to prove any of these hypotheses as it is impossible to determine exactly when HPV virus was transmitted in any particular case and for how long it has been present. This can be very confusing for those with genital warts as no definite answers can be given as to when they became infected. This can be distressing and put considerable strain on relationships.

FOLLOW-UP

Follow-up is very important after a diagnosis of genital warts. It almost always takes more than one treatment for the warts to disappear and frequent visits to the clinic may be necessary. Patients are encouraged to bring their partners to the clinic to be examined for any sign of genital warts and treated accordingly.

While the warts are still present it is advised that sexual contact ceases. Sometimes treatment can be prolonged and this can put strain on the strongest relationships, so, more realistically in these cases, it is advised that condoms are used for sexual intercourse until the warts are gone.

Individuals with genital warts often experience anxiety about transmitting the virus and confusion as to where and when it was contracted. Moreover, the necessary frequent visits to the GUM clinic can cause problems in other areas of their life. It may be very difficult for individuals to attend clinic for treatment on a regular basis, especially if they are working and are unwilling to tell their employer the reason for their absence. Williams (1991) demonstrated this in a study of time taken out of work to attend for wart treatment. He showed that women were more likely than men to disclose the true reason for their absence to their employer.

Often women are very worried that the wart virus infection will lead to cervical cancer. They need regular cervical smear testing and in many cases colposcopy in order to monitor the situation. They should be reassured that the risk is very small and is dependent on many other co-factors.

All these fears can lead to a reduced sex drive and negative attitude to their partner and, in turn to sexual problems within the relationship. These problems should be borne in mind when nursing such individuals, as they may need to share these fears and to be given reassurance. They may need referral to a psychologist in order to work through their fears.

NURSE-LED MANAGEMENT OF GENITAL WART TREATMENT

In many GUM clinics the management of genital wart treatment is the responsibility of nurses. As the treatment of this condition can be complex the nurse will call upon many skills in order to treat the condition and to care for the individual's emotional and psychological needs.

A diagnosis of genital warts is traumatic in itself and initially much of the nurse's time may be spent explaining the causes and consequences of the condition. Women in particular have many concerns about the effect of HPV on the cervix and about the behaviour of genital warts during pregnancy. Patients need reassurance about issues of transmission and recurrence of the infection. The nurse needs to be knowledgeable in all aspects of sexual health in order to advise and counsel individuals effectively. When genital warts are particularly persistent it is a difficult task to help each patient remain optimistic throughout the course of treatment. In addition wart treatment can be painful – another reason for the nurse's support and reassurance.

The physical treatment of genital warts requires the nurse to call upon her skills of assessment and evaluation. It is useful for one nurse to be the lead nurse for each individual requiring wart treatment – a good example of the usefulness of the named-nurse concept. This ensures consistency and allows a relationship between nurse and patient to form for the duration of the treatment. Once medical diagnosis of genital warts has been made, the doctor will often take advice from the nurse about the choice of treatment. Once the treatment is decided, the regime will begin with either the nurse or the doctor applying the initial treatment, and then the nurse will apply subsequent treatments – in accordance with the clinic's protocol.

At each visit for treatment the nurse must clearly and accurately document treatment interventions, any improvement seen and any other observations. Many different methods to ensure consistency are used in GUM clinics. Wart treatment charts are popular: printed diagrams on which the sites of warts are indicated at each visit. This can be compared to the use of photographs by district nurses to monitor the improvement of leg ulcers. Obviously the use of photographs at each visit for genital wart treatment may be unacceptable but the correct use of wart charts can prove as effective. In some clinics, nursing care plans are used for the duration of treatment.

For a prolonged course of wart treatment, guidelines should be established on the duration of use of each different treatment and at which points the process will be reviewed by a doctor. Many clinics follow the *Guidelines for Good Practice* (Genito-Urinary Nurses Association, 1995), whereby a set number of applications of a particular treatment are recommended before the doctor's review. On the doctor's advice the treatment may be changed or the same treatment continued. A growing number of nurse practitioners are taking over the role of reviewer and the responsibility for prescribing wart treatment. The management of genital warts differs from clinic to clinic; in some places it has been shown to be unselective and poorly monitored (Reynolds *et al.*, 1993). It is suggested that genital wart treatment protocols should provide a framework for auditing treatment and maintaining standards.

The treatment of genital warts is a good example of the way in which the multidisciplinary team can work together, each discipline contributing their own expertise in order to achieve a successful result. It is an area where nurses can demonstrate their knowledge and practical skills to their full potential, and where nurses have an ideal opportunity for audit and research.

GLOSSARY

Colposcopy	Optical examination of the vagina and cervix
Immunofluorescence	The detection of antigenic material by microscopically observing the antibodies that have become attached to it
Keratin	A hard waterproof protein occurring in horny tissue such as hair, nails and the outer layers of the skin
Meatoscopy	Optical examination of the opening of the male urethra
Neoplasia	The process of tumour formation
Polymerase chain reaction	DNA is separated into two strands, primers are attached and an enzyme, DNA polymerase, used to make a template for further strands. Large numbers of copies of any sequence of DNA can be rapidly produced in this way.
Vacuolated	Cells with a small clear region in the cytoplasm, sometimes surrounded by a membrane. Vacuoles can be used to store cell products or for excretion.

REFERENCES

Birley, H.D.L.. Luzzi, G.A., Walker, M.M. *et al.* (1994) The association of human papillomavirus infection with balanoposthitis: a description of five cases with proposals for treatment. *International Journal of STD and AIDS*, **5**(2), 139–41.

Department of Health (1995) *Statistical Bulletin: Sexually Transmitted Diseases, England 1994*. Bulletin 1995/16.

Genito-Urinary Nurses Association (1995) Wart treatments, in *Guidelines for Good Practice*, GUNA.

Gross, G., Jablonska, S., Pfister, H. and Stegner, H.E. (1990) *Genital Papillomavirus Infections: Modern Diagnosis and Treatment*, Springer-Verlag, Berlin/Heidelberg.

Handley, J., Lawther, H., Horner, T. *et al.* (1992) Ten year follow-up study of women presenting to a genitourinary medicine clinic with anogenital warts. *International Journal of STD and AIDS*, **3**(1), 28–32.

Kinghorn, G.R., McMillan, A., Mulcahy, F. *et al.* (1993) An open, comparative study of the efficacy of 0.5% podophyllotoxin solution and 25% podophyllin solution in the treatment of condylomata acuminata in males and females. *International Journal of STD and AIDS*, **4**(4), 194–99.

Law, C., Merianos, A., Thompson, C. *et al.* (1991) Manifestations of anogenital HPV infection in the male partners of women with anogenital warts and/or abnormal cervical smears. *International Journal of STD and AIDS*, **2**(3), 188–94.

Nieminen, P., Koskimies, A.I. and Paavonen, J. (1991) Human papillomavirus DNA is not transmitted by semen. *International Journal of STD and AIDS*, **2**(3), 207–8.

Oriel, J.D. (1988) Anogenital papillomavirus infection in children. *British Medical Journal*, **296**, 1484–5.

Reynolds, M., Murphy, M., Waugh, M.A. and Lacey, C.J.N. (1993) An audit of treatment of genital warts: opening the feedback loop. *International Journal of STD and AIDS*, **4**(4), 226–31.

Sand Petersen, C., Agner, T., Ottevanger, V. *et al.* (1995) A single blind study of podophyllotoxin cream 0.5% and podophyllotoxin solution 0.5% in male patients with genital warts. *Genitourinary Medicine*, **71**(6), 391–2.

Thin, R.N. (1992) Meatoscopy: a simple technique to examine the distal anterior urethra in men. *International Journal of STD and AIDS*, **3**(1), 21–3.

Wikstrom, A., Lidbrink, P., Johansson, M. and Von Krogh, G. (1991) Penile human papillomavirus carriage among men attending Swedish STD clinics. *International Journal of STD and AIDS*, **2**(2), 105–9.

Williams, N.R. (1991) Absence from work due to treatment for genital warts. *Journal of Social and Occupational Medicine*, **41**, 117–18.

Genital herpes

OBJECTIVES

1. To explain the aetiology of *Herpes simplex* virus (HSV) infection.
2. To state the modes of transmission of HSV.
3. To recognize the signs and symptoms of genital herpes infection.
4. To describe the complications of HSV infection.
5. To state the diagnostic methods associated with HSV and, in particular, with genital herpes infection.
6. To explain the management of genital herpes infection.
7. To recognize the importance of follow-up for individuals with genital herpes infection.

SUMMARY

Genital herpes is a relatively common sexually transmitted infection caused by *Herpes simplex* virus 1 (HSV-1) and *Herpes simplex* virus 2 (HSV-2). It can occur in most parts of the anogenital region. There is usually an initial primary attack and it often recurs. It is painful and debilitating, causing systemic illness as well as genital symptoms.

This chapter describes the aetiology of genital herpes infection, the transmission of the causative organism and its manifestations. This includes discussion of both primary and recurrent genital herpes infection. Diagnostic methods are explored and the management of genital herpes is described. The importance of follow-up is discussed, along with the nurse's role within that.

EPIDEMIOLOGY

The Department of Health (1995) reported an upward trend in cases of genital herpes infection in England since 1987, from 16,669 in that year to 26,805 in 1994. Most of this increase occurred in women, who now account for 59% of all cases of first-attack genital herpes. Recurrent attacks accounted for 11,458 cases in 1994. Among the men approximately 5% of cases were acquired through homosexual contact.

If the figures are analysed separately according to age categories it appears that the majority of cases of first-attack genital herpes occur in the 20–34 age group. However, a significant number of cases were recorded in the under 16 (125) and 16–19 (1,862) age groups, hence implications for the effectiveness of sex education for young people.

HSV-2 appears to be much less prevalent than HSV-1, although data regarding this are not available from the KC60 reports obtained from GUM clinics.

MICROBIOLOGY

Herpes simplex virus has been recognized since the early twentieth century. The name 'herpes' is derived from a Greek word meaning 'to creep'. Herpes viruses are responsible for a range of different diseases:

- HSV-1 and HSV-2 cause cold sores and genital herpes.
- *Varicella zoster* causes chicken pox and shingles.
- Epstein–Barr causes infectious mononucleosis and possibly chronic fatigue syndrome.
- Human herpes 6 can cause mononucleosis-type syndromes and lymphadenopathy. It may be a co-factor in the pathogenesis of AIDS.
- Cytomegalovirus — a common organism which becomes pathogenic, particularly in immunocompromised individuals.

The herpes viruses are large and enveloped and contain a double strand of DNA. This core of DNA is surrounded by a capsid, in turn enclosed by a glycoprotein-containing envelope. Viral proteins and enzymes are contained between these layers.

HSV can infect most types of human cells, causing lytic infections of the fibroblast and epithelial cells whereby the virus takes over the metabolic machinery of the cell. Latent infections of neurons also occur.

Entry into the host cell is achieved mainly by fusion of the HSV membrane and the host cell surface membrane. However, virions can also gain entry by endocytosis. The viral nucleocapsid is then released into the host cytoplasm. Once inside the cell the nucleocapsid fuses with the nuclear membrane of the host cell and transcription and replication of the nuclear material begin. The virus cannot replicate outside the host cell. The viral DNA fuses with the host's DNA and replicates along with it. The virus also delivers a viral encoded protein kinase and a transcriptional regulatory protein into the host cell. These help to initiate infection.

Replication of the virus within the host cell is complex and proceeds in three phases (Figure 12.1):

1. Immediate early: early proteins are synthesized, which are used for subsequent viral protein and nucleic acid synthesis.
2. Early: more specific proteins, such as enzymes, are synthesized.
3. Late: structural proteins are synthesized.

During a latent infection, replication does not proceed beyond the immediate early stage. Latent infection does not damage the host neurons at all. Once the early and late stages of replication are completed, the numerous new viral particles are expelled from the cell by exocytosis or cell lysis. This is when active infection begins. HSV usually causes a local infection, depending on its mode of spread.

Humoral and cellular immunity are important for the control of HSV in the body. Antibodies to the virus neutralize the extracellular virus and limit its spread. However, the antibodies can be evaded by direct spread from cell to cell and by latent infection of the neuron. In this case, cell-mediated immunity is needed to control and resolve the infection or the HSV infection may disseminate to the brain. The course of the immunological response is different in the primary attack and in recurrences.

During the initial attack, natural killer cells and interferon both work to limit the progress of the infection. Macrophages present viral antigens to the CD4 helper T cells and B cells to initiate antibody production. This immunological activity, as well as helping resolve the infection, can exacerbate the symptoms of the initial inflammatory responses. This results in swelling and soreness of the affected area.

Recurrent infections of HSV are usually less severe, more localized and of a much shorter duration. The virus reactivates despite the presence of antibody but the presence of local immunity helps resolve the infection quickly. The cause of recurrences is not clearly understood – a subject discussed later in the chapter.

If a person carries antibodies to HSV-1 and contracts HSV-2, the symptoms and clinical course are usually milder due to antibodies recognizing the herpes virus and acting against it. It was believed that genital herpes was usually caused by HSV-2 and herpes on the mouth, or 'cold sores', was caused by HSV-1. More recently it has been demonstrated that a far higher proportion of cases of genital herpes are caused by HSV-1 than was previously thought.

In men genital herpes is predominantly caused by HSV-2, although milder cases of genital herpes caused by HSV-1 have been misdiagnosed, as non-specific balanitis for example. In women, cases of genital herpes are now thought to be caused in equal numbers by HSV-1 and HSV-2 (Woolley and Kudesia, 1990).

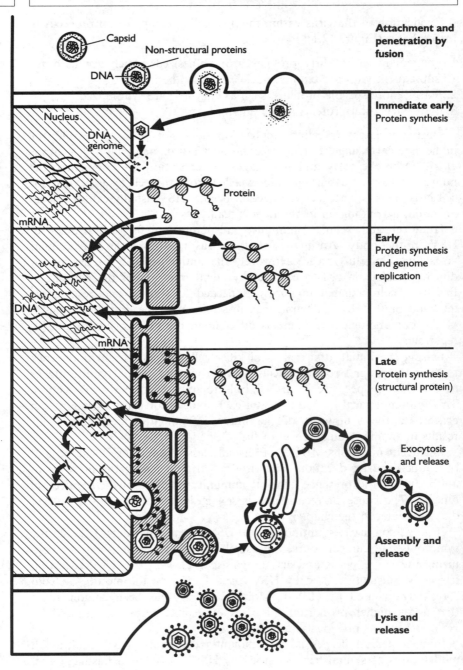

Figure 12.1 Replication of *Herpes simplex* virus.

Oral HSV-1 is common in children whereas HSV-2 is generally transmitted later when the individual becomes sexually active.

TRANSMISSION

There are several ways in which genital herpes can be transmitted.

Sexual intercourse

Genital herpes is transmitted through sexual contact with a person carrying the virus. The virus enters the body through the mucosal membrane or through breaks in the skin. There may be no viral replication at that site. If replication occurs, vesicular lesions appear. The virus undergoes replication at the base of the lesion and the fluid produced contains the infectious virions. The lesion will heal without a scar and the virus spreads up to the innervating neuron. A latent infection is established here. It has been observed that HSV-2 recurs more frequently on a sacral site than does HSV-1. This suggests that each virus type has adapted specifically to one local area.

HSV-1 is transmitted through saliva and it is therefore possible to transmit this virus to the genital area through orogenital sex. A small percentage of women with genital herpes may shed the virus from the cervix without any visible lesions. A smaller number of men also appear to shed the virus while they are asymptomatic. This may occur unnoticed for several reasons (Bowman *et al.*, 1990):

- The person may be unaware of the ulcers.
- The ulcers may be microscopic.
- The ulcers may be concealed, e.g. on the cervix.
- Other symptoms may mask the HSV, e.g. candidiasis.

This may help to explain why the sexual partner of someone with a primary attack of genital herpes appears to have no evidence or history of the disease. It is important to emphasize, however, that asymptomatic viral shedding appears to occur in only a small number of people and the actual rate of transmission by this means has yet to be established.

In pregnancy

Herpes simplex virus can be transmitted to the fetus in a number of ways:

- transplacentally
- during delivery
- postnatally

If transplacental infection occurs before the twentieth week of pregnancy, spontaneous abortion can occur. After 20 weeks' gestation the main risk to the fetus is the passage through the birth canal if the mother has a primary infection, as large amounts of virus may be shed from her cervix. There is less risk from a mother with recurrent disease as her circulating antibodies will afford some degree of protection. Other sources of infection to the neonate may include:

- the mother's infected breast
- iatrogenic, e.g. fetal scalp electrodes or infection from staff members

If the mother has a primary attack of genital herpes at the time of delivery, caesarean section is considered. If it is known that the mother is at risk of genital HSV infection because her partner has recurrent disease, she must be examined carefully at each antenatal visit and at delivery.

Auto-infection

It is possible for an individual to infect themselves in the genital area from a herpes lesion on the mouth and vice versa. This is more likely during a primary attack than in recurrence, as in the latter case the body will have produced antibodies preventing infection at other sites. In addition HSV can be transmitted from a genital lesion to the cornea. It is especially important that strict attention is paid to hand washing during an attack. HSV-2 infection in the eye can be serious and blindness can result if the infection is not treated.

It has been suggested that HSV may be transmitted by fomites such as wet towels. Although theoretically possible, this is highly unlikely as it is difficult for the virus to survive outside the body for long periods.

SIGNS AND SYMPTOMS

The signs and symptoms differ for primary and recurrent attacks.

Primary attack

The incubation period for HSV-2 with no previous infection of HSV-1 or HSV-2 is usually 2–20 days. However, retrospective clinical surveys have shown that the incubation period can be as long as 49 days (Thin, 1991). The symptoms of infection with HSV-2 are milder if the individual already has antibodies to HSV-1.

The resulting primary lesions begin as small vesicles, which join to form larger ulcerative lesions after about five days. These lesions then crust over and eventually resolve within 2–4 weeks. There may be many lesions and they are usually extremely painful.

In men the lesions are commonly found in the following anatomical locations:

- shaft of the penis
- glans of the penis
- urethra, causing dysuria
- anal and perianal areas

And in women:

- vulva
- vagina (less common)
- cervix
- perineal area
- inner thighs

Women may also experience itching and vaginal discharge. In both sexes HSV lesions may occur extragenitally, most commonly on the thighs, buttocks and suprapubic region. Several explanations are suggested (Mindel, Carney and Williams, 1990):

- sexual contact
- auto-inoculation
- intra-neural spread (along nerve pathways to new sites)

In both sexes a primary infection may be accompanied by the following symptoms:

- fever
- malaise
- myalgia
- dysuria
- inguinal adenitis
- sacral anaesthesia
- impotence
- urinary retention
- constipation

Urinary retention can be due to sacral nerve involvement, particularly with anal or perianal lesions, or extreme pain on passing urine. This can result in hospital admission. Women may find it easier to urinate in a warm bath.

Recurrent attack

Recurrent attacks of genital herpes result from the reactivation of the latent virus in the sacral ganglion. The virus migrates along the nerve pathway, usually appearing in the same area on each recurrence. Recurrences are less severe and can be preceded by a recognizable prodrome of itching or tingling in the area. The vesicles usually appear in only one area and are mildly painful. They usually disappear within ten days. Some people may never experience a recurrence; others may have recurrences every 2–3 weeks.

The triggers of recurrent attacks of herpes are not clearly understood. Several factors seem to be influential:

- exposure of the affected area to ultraviolet light
- skin trauma of the affected area
- stress
- menstruation

Complications

Proctitis

This is common in homosexual men, causing fever, ano-rectal pain, inguinal adenopathy, constipation, blood in faeces and rectal discharge. Herpes lesions can be seen on the perineum and anus and ulceration of the distal rectum can result.

Herpetic pharyngitis

This usually results from HSV contracted during oral sex. Individuals will experience severe soreness in the throat, malaise, fever and headache. The condition often goes undiagnosed.

Meningitis

This is not uncommon, particularly in women and occurs within ten days of infection with HSV-2. Symptoms can be severe but usually resolve quickly.

Herpes encephalitis

This usually occurs with HSV-1 but in infants HSV-2 is more likely. The condition is usually fatal and can occur in a primary attack or in recurrence. The virus migrates down the olfactory nerve into the brain, where it destroys the cells and causes necrosis.

HSV in the immunocompromised

Anogenital herpes can be particularly severe in the immunocompromised, e.g. those with HIV. There is a risk of viraemia and dissemination.

Eczema herpeticum

Existing eczema may become infected with HSV, causing extensive herpetic lesions which can be severe and prolonged.

Pregnancy and the newborn

HSV-2 can be acquired *in utero* but more often during passage through the birth canal, particularly when there is prolonged contact with the cervix. It is especially dangerous when there is a primary genital attack at the time of the birth. The significance of asymptomatic viral shedding in this case has not as yet been established. Transmission of HSV to the neonate can be life threatening, involving the lungs, liver and central nervous system and often resulting in herpes encephalitis.

In addition to the above complications of HSV infection, there has been some research into the possibility of a link between HSV-2 infection and the development of cervical cancer. This theory remains unproven but it is advisable that women with genital herpes should have regular cervical smear testing.

DIAGNOSIS

Initial diagnosis of genital herpes infection is made on clinical presentation, for it is important to commence treatment promptly, particularly with a primary attack. Several techniques can be used to isolate HSV; these are discussed below.

Culture

This method is the most effective diagnostic test for acute HSV infections. Its success is dependent on the stage of the herpes lesion. The earlier the specimen is collected, the higher the rate of detection. A cotton-tipped swab is used to collect the vesicular fluid from the lesions and inoculated straight into the culture medium. In order to collect a satisfactory specimen the swab must be rubbed firmly over the lesion. It is important to warn the patient of this as it may be painful.

The culture must be promptly inoculated and incubated. *Herpes simplex* virus will produce a cytopathic effect on the culture cells in 1–3 days, whereby they become enlarged and balloonlike. Various techniques of chemical confirmation are performed if the culture is positive in order to eliminate contaminants.

During these tests, HSV typing can be achieved using monoclonal antibodies; HSV-1 and HSV-2 can be identified by differences in their growth characteristics.

Cytology/histology

This method relies on the detection of an infected cell from a suspected HSV lesion. Multinucleated giant cells may be seen on staining. This is not as sensitive as culture although it is quicker and cheaper. The main disadvantage with this technique is that HSV infection cannot be distinguished from *Varicella zoster* virus.

Fluorescent antibody techniques

Herpes simplex virus antigen can be seen in cells using immunofluorescence techniques. This technique is quicker than culture testing but is not as sensitive, especially in individuals who are asymptomatic. The method relies on a high virus titre in the specimen and having good quality specimens.

Serological procedures

This can provide evidence of primary HSV infection, but a rise in antibody does not usually accompany a recurrence so these procedures are useless in diagnosing recurrent HSV infection. One of the main uses for serology testing for HSV is to diagnose asymptomatic HSV infection. This is important in individuals who are immunosuppressed, who can be offered prophylactic antiviral therapy.

There is a clear need for research into improving the accuracy and sensitivity of serology testing methods. *Herpes simplex* virus can often be detected on a cervical smear test but this cannot be relied on for accurate diagnosis as it may be missed.

TREATMENT

There is no cure for genital herpes. However, there are preparations available that can alleviate symptoms and control recurrences. Aciclovir is a drug that acts specifically on cells infected with HSV and therefore has very few side effects. The drug is available in oral, topical and intravenous preparations. The recommended regime for outpatient treatment is:

For first episode HSV: 200 mg five times daily for five days.
For suppressing recurrences: 200 mg four times daily for two months.

There are variations in the dosages used for the suppression of recurrences. There is evidence that continuous oral use of acyclovir to control recurrences of genital herpes can help considerably with people who are experiencing emotional dysfunction (Carney *et al.*, 1993).

No serious side effects of long-term therapy have been noted and no resistance reported.

The topical preparation can shorten the duration of attacks if applied every four hours but it is less effective than the oral preparation. If the HSV attack is severe enough for the patient to be admitted into hospital the intravenous preparation is used to alleviate symptoms as soon as possible.

Acyclovir is not yet licensed for use in pregnancy, although it is used under medical supervision, yet there is no national policy concerning this. Treatment policies vary from centre to centre.

Other drugs have recently been shown to be effective against HSV. Famciclovir and valaciclovir are similar to acyclovir but they do not have to be taken as frequently, which may improve compliance and be more acceptable to patients. The recommended dosages are as follows:

Famciclovir

First episode HSV: 250 mg three times daily for five days.
Recurrence: 125 mg twice daily for five days.

Valaciclovir

First episode HSV: 500 mg twice daily for five days.
Recurrence: 500 mg twice daily for five days.

Neither of these drugs is currently licensed for use during pregnancy.

The management of genital herpes varies amongst GU physicians. Some reasons for this are as follows (Russell *et al.*, 1993):

- Recently trained physicians may not have developed a sense of the differences in severity of genital herpes; the experience of nurses is of assistance here.
- If physicians have developed their counselling skills sufficiently, this may enable them to support patients through recurrences without medication. But the expertise and support of nurses and health advisers are also very important.
- Some physicians may prescribe topical aciclovir, reserving the oral preparation for more severe attacks. This may be an established prescribing pattern among more experienced physicians. Topical aciclovir is now available over the counter.
- There are cost implications in the management of genital herpes. Oral aciclovir is very expensive and this fact will influence prescribing practice.

Alternative remedies have been suggested. Recent studies demonstrate the usefulness of natural forms of treatment. One such study shows that chemical compounds called flavonoids obtained from bees have anti-viral properties and significantly speeded up recovery from herpes attacks (Arne Ring, 1995). It is important for clients suffering from herpes to explore all available options in order to alleviate their symptoms as much as possible.

Several studies are currently in progress seeking an effective vaccination for herpes. Although there is no cure for herpes, several measures can be taken to relieve the symptoms:

- analgesia to relieve pain
- local anaesthetic preparations to reduce discomfort
- urinating in a warm bath to reduce the stinging pain of dysuria

FOLLOW-UP

Herpes can have severe physical and psychological effects on sufferers and their partners. Follow-up is important, especially for those who suffer recurrence of the symptoms. The nurse has an important role in meeting the individual's need for support and advice; a supportive relationship is formed if repeated visits to the clinic are required.

As well as causing physical discomfort and pain, herpes can cause much emotional and psychological upset, often putting considerable strain on relationships. Unfortunately there is still a stigma associated with herpes, which can affect self-esteem. In one study, 50% of people with recurrent genital HSV suffered from depression, 15% had suicidal thoughts and 10% avoided further sexual relationships (Chandiok, 1992).

Although most of the work on the psychological effects of herpes infection has been based on the study of individuals with recurrent herpes, the impact of a diagnosis of primary herpes must not be ignored. It appears that such a diagnosis places a severe emotional burden on those affected, although this may lessen in time if no recurrences are experienced (Carney et al., 1994). The psychological effects of herpes and other sexually transmitted infections are fully explored in Chapter 4.

Studies have highlighted the main concerns of individuals with herpes:

- fear of telling new sexual partners about the diagnosis
- fear of further intimate relationships
- fear of disclosing the diagnosis to family and friends
- concerns about transmission of the virus to sexual partners
- concerns about transmission of the virus during pregnancy

It appears that living with recurrent genital herpes has a more profound effect on women than on men. Women seem more likely to feel less desirable and less confident (Brookes, Haywood and Green, 1993).

Genital herpes is a complex condition with many possible manifestations and outcomes. It is difficult to reassure clients when there is so much uncertainty, therefore it is imperative that correct information and support are offered to enable those affected to cope and to adapt to living with the infection. Certain key issues should be discussed with the client:

- the possibility of recurrence
- the risk of infecting one's current partner
- the risk of infecting future partners
- herpes in pregnancy
- ways of minimizing recurrences

It may be helpful for the nurse or health adviser to talk to the client and their partner together about their fears and problems. It may also be helpful to encourage liaison with an appropriate support group such as the Herpes Viruses Association. It is important to emphasize that genital herpes is common; thus meeting other people suffering from similar problems may be beneficial. Educational materials such as videos and leaflets are also available and many people find these useful for both themselves and their partners.

Although there is no sure means of preventing herpes, certain measures are advised:

- learning to recognize prodromal symptoms
- avoiding sexual contact while prodromal symptoms or lesions are present
- use of condoms
- careful hygiene and hand washing to prevent auto-infection
- spermicides containing nonoxenol-9, which can inactivate herpes viruses

It is important to remember that individuals experiencing recurrent genital herpes often have very clear ideas about the causes of their recurrences. Their understanding of the disease may be very different from the nursing or medical understanding. It is therefore important to give clear information to the individual without dismissing their own ideas.

GLOSSARY

Adenitis   Inflammation of a lymph node or gland

Cytopathic   Pertaining to abnormal changes in cells

Fibroblast   Cell that generates the protein collagen

Kinase   An enzyme activator

Myalgia	Pain in the muscles
Prodrome	A sign or symptom that precedes the start of a disease and gives early warning
Transplacentally	Passing across the placenta
Vesicular	Relating to or containing vesicles
Viraemia	The presence of viruses in the blood

REFERENCES

Arne Ring, S. (1995) Antiviral complex of flavonoids from propolis in the treatment of herpes infections. *Journal of Alternative and Complementary Medicine*, **13**(1), 9–10.

Bowman, C.A., Woolley, P.D., Herman, S. *et al.* (1990) Asymptomatic herpes simplex virus shedding from the genital tract whilst on suppressive doses of oral acyclovir. *International Journal of STD and AIDS*, **1**(3), 174–7.

Brookes, J.L., Haywood, S. and Green, J. (1993) Adjustment to the psychological and social sequelae of recurrent genital herpes simplex infection. *Genitourinary Medicine*, **69**(5), 384–7.

Carney, O., Ross, E., Ikkos, G. and Mindel, A. (1993) The effect of suppressive oral aciclovir on the psychological morbidity associated with recurrent genital herpes. *Genitourinary Medicine*, **69**(6), 457–9.

Carney, O., Ross, E., Bunker, C. *et al.* (1994) A prospective study of the psychological impact on patients with a first episode of genital herpes. *Genitourinary Medicine*, **70**(1), 40–5.

Chandiok, S. (1992) The GP's role in the management of viral STDs. *Journal of Sexual Health*, **1**(1), 32–3.

Department of Health (1995) *Statistical Bulletin: Sexually Transmitted Diseases, England 1994.* Bulletin 1995/16.

Mindell, A., Carney, O. and Williams, P. (1990) Cutaneous herpes simplex infections. *Genitourinary Medicine*, **66**(1), 14–15.

Murray, P.R., Drew, W.L., Kobayashi, G.S. and Thompson, J.H. (1990) *Medical Microbiology*, Wolfe, USA, p. 503.

Russell, J.M., Cracknell, M., Barton, S.E. and Catalan, J. (1993) Management of genital herpes by genitourinary physicians. Does experience or doctor's gender influence clinical management? *Genitourinary Medicine*, **69**(2), 115–18.

Thin, R.N. (1991) Does first episode genital herpes have an incubation period? A clinical study. *International Journal of STD and AIDS*, **2**(4), 286–8.

Woolley, P.D. and Kudesia, G. (1990) Incidence of herpes simplex virus type-1 and type-2 from patients with primary (first-attack) genital herpes in Sheffield. *International Journal of STD and AIDS*, **1**(3), 184–6.

Vaginal infections | 13

OBJECTIVES

1. To describe the most common causes of vaginal discharge, both infective and non-infective.
2. To explain the microbiology, transmission, signs and symptoms, methods of detection, and treatment of *Trichomonas vaginalis* in women.
3. To recognize the significance of *Trichomonas vaginalis* in men.
4. To describe the microbiology, signs and symptoms, diagnosis and treatment of bacterial vaginosis.
5. To discuss the theories about the transmission and occurrence of bacterial vaginosis.
6. To explain the microbiology and main causes of genital candidiasis.
7. To recognize the methods of detection and main treatment regimes of the vaginal infections described.
8. To describe the non-infectious causes of vaginal discharge.

SUMMARY

This chapter describes the microbiology, transmission, symptomology, diagnosis and treatment of common vaginal infections. The infections described in this chapter are:

- *Trichomonas vaginalis*
- anaerobic vaginosis
- candidiasis

THE SIGNIFICANCE OF VAGINAL DISCHARGE

It would be erroneous to suggest that all vaginal discharge indicates infection. The vagina naturally produces secretions for lubrication and protec-

Table 13.1 Changes in secretions throughout the menstrual cycle

Quality of mucus measured	Scoring points			
	0	1	2	3
Volume	None	Scanty	Dribbling	Cascade
Spinnbarkeit	None	<3 cm	<8 cm	<8 cm
Ferning	None	Slight	Partial	Complete
Cervix	Closed; pale pink mucosa		Partially open	Gaping os; hyperaemic mucosa

Note: Day 0 = ovulation; on days –1, 0 and +1 the score should be over 8.

tion against infection. The amount and appearance of these secretions varies from woman to woman and alters during the menstrual cycle (see Table 13.1). Just before ovulation the vaginal mucus appears clear and stringy, whereas at ovulation it becomes thin and increases in volume. The contraceptive pill and pregnancy can also increase the amount of vaginal discharge. This can cause confusion, especially in women who are not familiar with the anatomy and physiology of their own bodies.

There are other causes of vaginal discharge not associated with infection. These include allergies to rubber, latex or soaps. Moreover, foreign bodies such as a retained tampon can cause a profuse malodorous discharge. In order to establish quickly the cause of vaginal discharge it is important to take a careful history of symptoms and to perform a thorough examination.

TRICHOMONAS VAGINALIS

Epidemiology

The Department of Health (1995) reported that the number of new cases of *Trichomonas vaginalis* seen in GUM clinics in England fell between 1984 and 1994 from 16,751 to 5,559. In 1994 only 323 of the new cases were men.

Microbiology

Trichomonas vaginalis is a protozoan responsible for urogenital infections in women and to a much lesser extent in men. The organism is round or oval in shape, 10–20 μm wide and has four flagella and an undulating

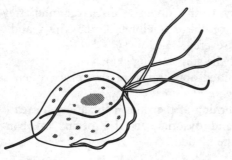

Figure 13.1 Diagram of *Trichomonas vaginalis*.

membrane used for movement (See Figure 13.1). It reproduces by binary fission and is anaerobic. Carbohydrate is the main source of energy, mainly glycogen in the cells of the vaginal mucosa.

Transmission

Trichomonas vaginalis in adults is sexually transmitted. The main evidence for this is the frequency with which it is isolated along with other sexually transmitted infections such as gonorrhoea. In addition, contact tracing can sometimes identify a chain of infection. This is substantiated by research showing a high prevalence of *Trichomonas vaginalis* among male sexual contacts of infected women (Krieger *et al.*, 1993b).

The organism has been known to survive outside the body for up to 24 hours in moist environments. However, transmission by fomites such as towels is rare and the results of studies on this tend to be inconclusive. There are some reported cases of female infants becoming infected during passage through the birth canal of infected mothers, resulting in vulvitis in the infant.

Signs and symptoms

Women

The incubation period of the organism is difficult to ascertain. It is estimated to be 3–21 days but usually takes up to a week to appear. This ambiguity can be attributed to the fact that up to 50% of women remain asymptomatic or exhibit only very mild symptoms.

Symptomatic cases of *Trichomonas vaginalis* are usually characterized by:

- profuse watery, frothy, offensive discharge often grey/green in colour;
- inflammation of the epithelium of the vulva and vagina, which can sometimes be severe;
- excoriation of the surrounding skin;
- a reddened, pitted appearance of the cervix, often called a 'strawberry cervix';
- itching and burning of the skin in the affected area;
- dyspareunia and dysuria can also occur, involving the urethra and occasionally the bladder.

Symptoms can worsen during or after menstruation and during pregnancy.

Men

Although *Trichomonas vaginalis* is a well recognized infection of sexually active women, its significance in men has yet to be established. Its prevalence in male sexual contacts of infected women is as much as 22% (Krieger *et al.*, 1993a). The low rate of detection of this organism in men is mainly due to the fact that most male sexual contacts of affected women are asymptomatic. In addition to this, diagnostic methods for males are not ideal or practical, semen samples proving the most effective for culture (Krieger *et al.*, 1993a).

Although many men with *Trichomonas vaginalis* remain asymptomatic, it has been observed that mild urethral discharge is the most common manifestation (Krieger *et al.*, 1993b). This may be significant in cases of men complaining of urethral symptoms but with no discharge on examination or no other cause (e.g. *Chlamydia trachomatis*) detected. It has also been noted that, although asymptomatic, some men remain carriers of *Trichomonas vaginalis* for long periods of time. This has implications for men who are sexually active during this time, especially those with more than one partner. It has also been observed that trichomonads can survive in semen for up to 24 hours, which provides an effective vehicle for transmission (Daly *et al.*, 1989).

In a recent study 35% of untreated men who were re-evaluated had experienced spontaneous resolution (Krieger *et al.*, 1993a). It is suggested that high concentrations of zinc and other inhibitory substances in secretions from the prostate gland may protect the male urogenital tract against organisms such as *Trichomonas vaginalis*.

Diagnosis

There are several methods of diagnosis for *Trichomonas vaginalis*. A specimen of vaginal discharge is taken from the posterior vaginal fornix. Although the organism can also be isolated from cervical specimens the yield from the vaginal specimen is superior (Boeke, Dekker and Peer-booms, 1993).

In men the specimen is taken from the urethra. Specimens can be obtained from urine sediment. These are no more effective than urethral specimens but are more time consuming to obtain.

Methods of detection

Saline wet mount

A sample from the vagina (or urethra in men) is mixed with a drop of saline on a microscope slide and covered with a cover slip. The slide is then scrutinized under dark-field or reduced light microscopy under high power ($\times 1000$). The trichomonads can be recognized from the characteristic jerky movement as they use their flagella. This method has proved adequate for routine diagnosis, although the degree of success is affected by the experience of the microscopist, the number of organisms present and the promptness of reading the slide.

Culture

The specimen is added to Stuart's or Amies' medium and incubated at 37°C for 48 hours. This method has been found to be extremely effective in the diagnosis of this organism. The main disadvantage, however, is the length of time needed for culture. In a clinic situation, speed of diagnosis is imperative.

Trichomonas vaginalis can also be detected on the Papanicolaou cervical smear; however, this cannot be relied on for diagnostic purposes and is usually detected incidentally.

It is very important to perform a full screen for other sexually transmitted infections, as *Trichomonas vaginalis* is sometimes found coexisting with other organisms.

Treatment

The universal drug of choice for the treatment of trichomoniasis is metronidazole. A variety of regimes are used, most commonly:

- 200 mg twice a day for five days.
- Sometimes a single dose of 2 g is preferred for convenience and assurance of compliance.

Ideally, male and female partners are treated to eliminate reinfection.

Metronidazole therapy appears to be very effective, with a cure rate of over 90%. In some cases, however, the infection persists. This may be due to incomplete absorption of the drug or its inactivation by other microorganisms such as Group B streptococcus. In very resistant cases other treatments may be used, such as clotrimazole pessaries.

Metronidazole must be used with caution in the first trimester of pregnancy. Laboratory studies have shown a teratogenic effect in animals at high doses. It should also be avoided during lactation.

Follow-up

A follow-up visit is necessary in order to monitor the effectiveness of the treatment. On this visit, repeat tests for *Trichomonas vaginalis* are performed, often by the nursing staff, and there is the opportunity to discuss the results of screening tests and to advise on future sexual health. These discussions allow nurses to explore the issues comprehensively with the client.

In women with recurrent trichomoniasis, contact tracing of partners may be beneficial and should be encouraged. Policies on contact tracing for trichomoniasis vary between GUM clinics but it is important for women to recognize their partner's role and responsibility in this situation. It is helpful for partners to be examined, treated and advised on general issues of sexual health. The use of condoms is advised to minimize the chances of reinfection with *Trichomonas vaginalis* and for the promotion of general sexual health.

BACTERIAL VAGINOSIS

Bacterial vaginosis is also known as 'gardnerella' or 'anaerobic vaginosis'.

Epidemiology

The Department of Health (1995) has collected data on the incidence of bacterial vaginosis and balanitis since 1989. From 1989 to 1994 the number of reported cases rose from 36,293 to 53,894. Among women the number of reported cases increased from 34,144 to 41,734. In men the number of reported cases of balanitis also increased quite significantly, from 2,149 to 12,160. These figures show that, although they are not considered sexually transmitted infections, bacterial vaginosis and balanitis in men are being diagnosed with increasing frequency in GUM clinics in England.

Microbiology

Bacterial vaginosis is caused by several different types of bacteria, with some or all present at the same time. The most common microorganisms associated with this condition are:

- *Gardnerella vaginalis*
- *Mycoplasma hominis*
- *Mobiluncus*
- *Bacteroides*
- miscellaneous aerobes

All these bacteria can be found as commensals in the vagina, causing symptoms only when the lactobacilli are so reduced in number that other species are able to flourish. The cause of this is largely unknown, although some women notice symptoms at certain times in their menstrual cycle, which suggests hormonal influences. In support of this theory is the observation that bacterial vaginosis rarely seems to appear in postmenopausal women.

Gardnerella vaginalis is a facultative anaerobe exhibiting both Gram-positive and Gram-negative characteristics. It is non-motile, non-spore-forming and grows slowly in the presence of carbon dioxide.

Transmission

It has been difficult to establish the significance of bacterial vaginosis as a sexually transmitted infection. *Gardnerella vaginalis* has been isolated from the urethra of male partners and there is some evidence to suggest that some of the bacteria present in bacterial vaginosis cause symptoms of non-gonoccocal urethritis (Woolley *et al.*, 1990).

The recurrence rates of bacterial vaginosis in women whose partners remain untreated are not significantly different from those whose partners have been treated (Moi *et al.*, 1989; Larsson, 1992). The discovery of previously unknown bacteria may solve the mystery of bacterial vaginosis.

Other risk factors for the transmission of bacterial vaginosis have been suggested but none of these has been substantiated. They include:

- a previous history of *Trichomonas vaginalis*
- use of intrauterine devices for contraception
- oral contraceptives

The use of some soaps and detergents in the vulval area may cause symptoms in some women and should be discouraged.

There is some suggestion that bacterial vaginosis is associated with both gonoccocal and chlamydial infections in women and also seems more prevalent when vaginal or urethral inflammation is present (Moi, 1990). There is no doubt, however, that, whether sexually transmitted or otherwise, this is one of the commonest causes of vaginal discharge and thus a common diagnosis of women attending GUM clinics in the United Kingdom.

Signs and symptoms

Vaginal discharge is the most common manifestation. This is sometimes described as frothy and fishy, the smell often noticeable after sexual intercourse. Itching is also described but soreness of the vulva or vagina is not a recognized feature. There is some evidence that this condition may be associated with pre-term birth and low-birthweight babies; it is recommended that pregnant women should be screened and treated for this and other infections to prevent complications (Hauth *et al.*, 1995). Rarely, other complications are associated with this condition, in particular, bacteraemia and infection of the neonate.

Diagnosis

In 1983 a clinical diagnostic criterion was proposed by Amsel and colleagues. If three of four particular characteristics were observed, bacterial vaginosis could be diagnosed. These characteristics are:

1. The presence of the discharge associated with this condition.
2. The presence of clue cells on a wet or Gram stained slide. Clue cells appear as epithelial cells coated with numerous bacteria, often described as a 'salt and pepper' effect. It must be noted that clue cells can also be detected in asymptomatic women with no signs or symptoms of bacterial vaginosis.
3. A positive amine test. If a drop of 10% potassium hydroxide is added to the wet preparation a characteristic fishy odour can be detected. Amines are in a salt form at the normal vaginal pH of 4.5. If potassium hydroxide is added the amines are converted to a base form and then give off the characteristic odour as described.
4. A vaginal pH of more than 4.5. Care must be taken when measuring the pH as this can be affected by semen, blood or cervical mucus.

More recent work has suggested that a combination of the identification of clue cells and one other of these methods of detection is sufficient for the accurate diagnosis of bacterial vaginosis (Christiano *et al.*, 1989).

According to the above criteria it is possible to diagnose bacterial vaginosis in the absence of clue cells, provided the other criteria are met. This, however, can lead to confusion as there is evidence of some allergies to condoms and spermicides which appear to mimic the symptoms of this condition (Haye and Mandal, 1990).

Microscopy

The presence of bacterial vaginosis in a specimen of vaginal discharge can be detected on a wet preparation or a Gram stained slide observed at high magnification (× 1000). Under the wet preparation using dark-ground illumination, clue cells are seen. The epithelial cells do not have clear borders as normal but appear irregular and are coated with bacteria such as *Gardnerella vaginalis*. Light-field microscopy can also be used for this purpose. A similar appearance is seen on the Gram stained slide. Bacteria cover the epithelial cells and there is an absence of lactobacilli and neutrophils. The Gram stained slide method for the detection of clue cells is considered the quickest and most effective way to diagnose bacterial vaginosis (Thomason *et al.*, 1992).

It is possible to culture *Gardnerella vaginalis*, the most common medium being blood. This is rarely performed, because of the speed and effectiveness of the other diagnostic methods described.

Treatment

As with *Trichomonas vaginalis*, metronidazole is the drug of choice.

• The usual dosage is 400 mg twice daily for five days.
• A single dose of 2 g can also be used.

Metronidazole, however, is inactive against *Mycoplasma hominis*, which may explain the high recurrence of bacterial vaginosis. As yet unidentified bacteria may also contribute to this problem. Chlorhexidine pessaries have some effect as an alternative to metronidazole.

When bacterial vaginosis frequently recurs, male partners are often treated simultaneously. It is important for the wider issues of sexual health to be discussed. The use of condoms may be advised in order to minimize any sexual transmission of the causative bacteria and to promote general sexual health.

GENITAL CANDIDIASIS

This common condition is better known as 'thrush' and historically as 'monilia'. It can affect women of all ages but appears to be more common in sexually active women of child-bearing age.

Epidemiology

Candidiasis has consistently been one of the most common conditions diagnosed in GUM clinics in England for some time. The incidence of candidiasis in England has remained steady since 1984 (Department of Health, 1995). There were 64,787 new cases in 1994.

Among women a rise in incidence is reported between 1984 and 1994, from 47,535 cases to 55,539. In men the number of reported cases within the same ten years decreased from 12,133 to 9,248.

Microbiology

Genital candidiasis is caused by one of several fungi, the most common being *Candida albicans*. Others include *Torulopsis glabrata, C. tropicalis* and *C. parapsilosis*. *Candida albicans* takes the form of an oval spore which buds forming long threadlike filaments known as 'hyphae'. The cells of the hyphae elongate and are linked together like sausages. Unlike other yeasts, newly formed cells are not pinched off after budding but continue to grow.

Transmission

There is little evidence to suggest sexual transmission although some male partners of women with candidiasis may show symptoms. *Candida* spp. have been shown to be a major cause of balanitis and balanoposthitis in men, which often occur after sexual intercourse (Abdullah *et al.*, 1992). In women it is generally accepted that factors other than sexual transmission are more important, as described below (Hart, 1993).

Candida albicans can be found in many parts of the body including the colon, mouth, nails, rectum and vagina and cause no symptoms. It thrives in warm, moist environments, e.g. under the breasts in women.

Some women may experience one attack of vaginal candidiasis and some more frequent and chronic problems. Although in many cases a cause cannot be identified the following factors have been suggested:

1. Response to hormonal influences during the menstrual cycle and in pregnancy: it is thought that increased oestrogen levels at these times increase the glycogen levels in the vagina, which in turn reduces cell-mediated immunity, allowing the fungus to proliferate.
2. During the use of antibacterials: the use of antibiotics reduces the numbers of lactobacilli, thus altering the balance of natural flora in the vagina and precipitating candidiasis.
3. The role of oral contraceptives: a link has been suggested between candidiasis and the use of oral contraceptives. As the woman's cycle is dominated by progesterone when she is using the oral contraceptive, the vaginal epithelium fails to mature fully and may be less resistant to infection. There may also be a general reduction in immunity.
4. Trauma to the vagina, including from sexual intercourse.
5. The presence of diabetes mellitus: both vaginal candidiasis and candidal balanitis in men can be a sign of poorly controlled diabetes. An environment with an abundance of glucose is ideal for candidal growth.
6. Immunosuppression: candidiasis is common and often severe in people whose immune system is deficient, e.g. those with HIV.

7. When irritants are present: chemical irritants such as perfumed soap and other detergents can upset the balance of flora in the vagina.

For people experiencing more chronic candidiasis the causes are more difficult to identify. It has been suggested that the candidal spores may penetrate the vaginal wall more deeply in some people, causing frequent relapses as the epithelial cells are shed. And for some the perineum may be more heavily colonized with *Candida* from the rectum.

Signs and symptoms

Women

The most common symptoms of candidiasis are:

- itching of the vaginal and sometimes the perineal area
- thick, whitish, curdy discharge
- dysuria and dyspareunia in some cases.

Inflammation of the vulval area can occur; in some cases it is severe, with oedema of the labia and excoriation of the surrounding skin, sometimes extending down the thighs. The vaginal discharge will have a lower pH than the normal 4.5.

Men

Occasionally the male partners of women with candidiasis can experience itchiness and erythema of the glans and subpreputial area of the penis. Phimosis is rare. If the penis is circumcised, there may be red scaly patches on the glans, perhaps with some obvious fissuring. Urethral symptoms are not usually associated with *Candida*. In some men it is thought that a hypersensitivity reaction of the penis occurs when in contact with *Candida*. This may be mistaken for candidiasis itself.

Diagnosis

Specimens are taken from the vaginal walls in women and the affected areas in men. *Candida* can be isolated from cervical specimens but optimum results will be obtained from the vagina (Boeke, Dekker and Peerbooms, 1993). A wet preparation with a drop of saline can be used or the specimen can be Gram stained, in both cases for examination under a microscope. The spores and hyphae appear as Gram-positive and are very distinctive. In addition a sample of discharge is cultured on Sabouraud media containing chloramphenicol to inhibit bacterial growth. It is then incubated at 25°C, which inhibits bacterial growth.

Treatment

Clotrimazole pessaries and cream are most commonly used for the treatment of vaginal candidiasis. The dosages may vary from a single dose pessary of 500 mg to a three-dose regime of 200 mg. These preparations can now be bought over the counter at any pharmacy; however, it is advisable to attend a GUM clinic for several reasons:

- to have swab tests to confirm that candidiasis is the correct diagnosis;
- to exclude any other infections;
- to receive adequate follow-up to ensure the treatment is effective;
- to receive advice about prevention of further attacks and to discuss future sexual health.

Other drugs can be prescribed by a doctor, for example itraconazole, which is found to be equally effective but is more expensive and cannot be used in pregnancy or for breast-feeding mothers because animal studies have indicated toxicity. Systemic antifungals are not usually recommended for women who experience only occasional attacks. For women with more chronic problems a single-dose oral preparation is available, fluconazole 150 mg. This, being systemically absorbed, may be more effective in the deeper vaginal tissues and may reach the places topical antifungals do not. Unfortunately the oral preparation is not yet licensed for use in pregnancy. Drug resistance is not recognized in the treatment of candidiasis, thus recurrence is not related to this (Fong, Bannatyne and Wong, 1993).

In some cases of chronic candidiasis, suppressive therapy with clotrimazole is used with some success, in particular when dosages are timed to coincide with certain stages of the menstrual cycle.

Alternative therapies are popular in the treatment of candidiasis. These include live natural yoghurt put inside the vagina, which may help restore the lactobacilli to sufficient numbers to combat the candida. For women who are certain that their symptoms are caused by candida, various self-help methods can be effective:

- wearing cotton underwear;
- wearing stockings instead of tights;
- wearing skirts instead of trousers or jeans;
- refraining from using perfumed soaps and other detergents;
- when wiping the genital area after going to the toilet, using the front to back method.

It must be advised, however, that an initial assessment and examination in a GUM clinic will aid diagnosis and appropriate treatment. In addition any other infective or non-infective causes of symptoms can be eliminated. For men, application of clotrimazole cream to the affected area is usually sufficient. For men with suspected hypersensitivity reactions, 1% hydrocortisone cream is effective.

NON-SPECIFIC VAGINITIS

The menstrual cycle and other hormonal changes can affect the vaginal secretions. At the menopause some women may experience other symptoms such as:

- vaginal discharge
- vaginal dryness
- soreness
- bleeding
- urinary symptoms

The skin of the vagina and cervix may appear thin, and Gram-positive organisms are often detected. These symptoms are indicative of atrophic vaginitis due to a lack of oestrogen, which can be replaced by local preparations or orally. All infective causes must still be eliminated in these cases, however, and carcinoma of the cervix must also be ruled out by performing a cervical smear.

Vulval and vaginal conditions and infections can cause anxiety, particularly if recurrences are experienced. They can lead to a feeling of being sexually unhealthy and psychosexual problems may result. Such worries should be recognized and support and advice made readily available. Many women attend GUM clinics with non-infective skin conditions such as lichen sclerosus which have previously gone undiagnosed. Some GUM medics have a special interest in dermatology and may be experienced in the diagnosis and treatment of such conditions. Alternatively, referral to the appropriate speciality, usually dermatology, may be required.

GLOSSARY

Aerobe	An organism that can live and thrive only in the presence of oxygen
Anaerobe	A microorganism that can live and thrive in the absence of free oxygen. These are usually found in body cavities or wounds where the oxygen tension is low.
Balanitis	Inflammation of the glans penis
Balanoposthitis	Inflammation of the glans penis and prepuce (foreskin)

Binary fission	The multiplication of cells by division into two equal parts
Dyspareunia	Painful or difficult coitus for women
Dysuria	Difficulty or pain on passing urine
Facultative anaerobe	A microorganism that can live or grow with or without molecular oxygen
Fomite	An inanimate object or material on which disease-producing agents may be conveyed.
Phimosis	Constriction of the prepuce so that it cannot be drawn back over the glans penis
Protozoan	Single-celled, microscopic animal
Teratogenic	Property of an agent capable of causing physical defects in the developing embryo
Yeasts	Fungi of the genus *Saccharomyces*

REFERENCES

Abdullah, A.N., Drake, S.M., Wade, A.A.H. *et al.* (1992) Balanitis (balano-posthitis) in patients attending a department of genitourinary medicine. *International Journal of STD and AIDS*, **3**(2), 128–9.

Amsel, R., Totten, P.A., Spiegel, C.A. *et al.* (1983) Nonspecific vaginitis. Diagnostic criteria and microbial and epidemiologic associations. *American Journal of Medicine*, **74**, 14–22.

Boeke, A.J.P., Dekker, J.H. and Peerbooms, P.G.H. (1993) A comparison of yield from cervix versus vagina for culturing *Candida albicans* and *Trichomonas vaginalis*. *Genitourinary Medicine*, **69**(1), 41–3.

Christiano, L., Coffetti, N., Dalvai, G. *et al.* (1989) Bacterial vaginosis: prevalence in outpatients, association with some micro-organisms and laboratory indices. *Genitourinary Medicine*, **65**(6), 382–7.

Daly, J.J., Sherman, J.K., Green, L. and Hostetler, T.T. (1989) Survival of *Trichomonas vaginalis* in human semen. *Genitourinary Medicine*, **65**(2), 106–8.

Department of Health (1995) *Statistical Bulletin: Sexually Transmitted Diseases, England 1994*. Bulletin 1995/16.

Fong, I.W., Bannatyne, R.M.S. and Wong, P. (1993) Lack of in vitro resistance of *Candida albicans* to ketoconazole, itraconazole and clotrimazole in women treated for recurrent vaginal candidiasis. *Genitourinary Medicine*, **69**(1), 44–6.

Hart, G. (1993) Factors associated with trichomoniasis, candidiasis and bacterial vaginosis. *International Journal of STD and AIDS*, **4**(1), 21–5.

Haye, K.R. and Mandal, D. (1990) Allergic vaginitis mimicking bacterial vaginosis. *International Journal of STD and AIDS*, **1**(6), 440–2.

Hauth, J.C., Goldenberg, R.L., Andrews, W.W. *et al.* (1995) Reduced incidence of preterm delivery with metronidazole and erythromycin in women with bacterial vaginosis. *New England Journal of Medicine*, **333**, 1732–6.

Krieger, J.N., Verdon, M., Siegel, N. and Holmes, K.K. (1993a) Natural history of urogenital Trichomoniasis in men. *The Journal of Urology*, **149**, 1455–8.

Krieger, J.N., Jenny, C., Verdon, M. *et al.* (1993b) Clinical manifestations of Trichomonas in men. *Annals of Internal Medicine*, **118**(11), 844–9.

Larsson, P.-G. (1992) Treatment of bacterial vaginosis. *International Journal of STD and AIDS*, **3**(4), 239–47.

Moi, H., Erkkola, R., Jerve, F. *et al.* (1989) Should male consorts of women with bacterial vaginosis be treated? *Genitourinary Medicine*, **65**(4), 263–8.

Moi, H. (1990) Prevalence of bacterial vaginosis and its association with genital infections, inflammation, and contraceptive methods in women attending sexually transmitted disease and primary health clinics. *International Journal of STD and AIDS*, **1**(2), 86–94.

Thomason, J.L., Anderson, R.J., Gelbart, S.M. *et al.* (1992) Simplified Gram stain interpretive method for diagnosis of bacterial vaginosis. *American Journal of Obstetrics and Gynaecology*, **167**(1), 16–19.

Woolley, P.D., Kinghorn, G.R., Talbot, M.D. and Duerden, B.I. (1990) Microbiological flora in men with non-gonococcal urethritis with particular reference to anaerobic bacteria. *International Journal of STD and AIDS*, **1**(2), 122–5.

<table>
<tr><td>14</td><td># Molluscum contagiosum, pediculosis pubis and scabies</td></tr>
</table>

OBJECTIVES

1. To explain the aetiology of molluscum contagiosum, scabies and pediculosis pubis.
2. To describe the modes of transmission of these conditions.
3. To recognize the signs and symptoms associated with these conditions.
4. To explain the methods of diagnosis of these conditions.
5. To describe the treatment options for each of these conditions.

SUMMARY

This chapter describes molluscum contagiosum, a benign viral condition, and two infestations, scabies and pediculosis pubis. The epidemiology, aetiology and transmission of these conditions are considered, and methods of detection and treatment options are discussed.

MOLLUSCUM CONTAGIOSUM

Epidemiology

The numbers of cases of molluscum contagiosum are not available nationally as part of the annual figures for sexually transmitted infections.

Microbiology

The lesions of molluscum contagiosum are caused by an unclassified poxvirus. The diagnosis can be confirmed histologically by large eosinophilic cytoplasmic inclusions, called 'molluscum bodies', within epithelial cells, the samples obtained by biopsy specimens or the material expressed from the core of the lesion. The lesions are very distinctive and histological diagnosis is not usually necessary. The incubation period for molluscum contagiosum is 2–8 weeks.

Transmission

Molluscum contagiosum is not strictly a sexually transmitted infection, as there are other means of transmission. It is often seen in the genital area because it is spread by skin contact. It can also be transmitted by fomites, e.g. towels, which explains its appearance in children.

Signs and symptoms

There is usually more than one lesion and sometimes numerous lesions, most commonly on the genitals and trunk region of the body. The lesions begin as small papules and then become pearly nodules, which if squeezed produce a thick white discharge. They are often mistaken for warts. In individuals who are immunosuppressed, e.g. in HIV infection, the lesions may be large and numerous and often occur on the face and neck.

Diagnosis

Molluscum contagiosum is usually diagnosed by its distinctive clinical appearance. There is a dearth of research into the likelihood of other sexually transmitted diseases coexisting with molluscum contagiosum; however, a summary of several recent studies supports this theory and makes the following recommendations (Radcliffe, Daniels and Evans, 1991):

1. Patients presenting with molluscum contagiosum should be offered a full screen for sexually transmitted infections.
2. It is suggested that partners of those with molluscum contagiosum are screened in the same way.
3. Individuals presenting to GPs or other practitioners with molluscum contagiosum should be referred to a GUM clinic.

More research is needed to establish clearly the links between molluscum contagiosum and other sexually transmitted infections.

Treatment

It is known that, if left, the molluscum lesions will disappear spontaneously within 2–12 months due to acquired immune responses. Treatment is often requested, however, for aesthetic reasons, especially if the lesions are in the genital area. In addition, treatment is advisable to prevent further spread. The assessment and treatment of molluscum contagiosum is often carried out and monitored by nurses. The following are the two main treatments used in GUM clinics.

Phenol

This is applied carefully with a small needle or sharpened stick into the core of each lesion. It kills the virus and slowly the lesion will disappear. Phenol must be used with care as it can burn the surrounding skin.

Cryotherapy

This has become more popular recently. It is used in a similar way to the treatment of genital warts (see Chapter 11).

Follow-up

Follow-up is advisable in order to evaluate the effectiveness of treatment and to ensure there has been no reaction to the treatment itself. It also creates an opportunity to provide information and safe sex advice on the prevention of sexually transmitted infections.

SCABIES

Epidemiology

It is difficult to establish the exact number of cases of scabies seen in GUM clinics, because scabies and pediculosis pubis are reported collectively. In England the incidence of these two conditions has fallen by more than half from 12,226 cases in 1984 to 5,051 in 1994 (Department of Health, 1995). These two conditions are three times more common in men than women.

The incidence of scabies appears to be affected predominantly by socioeconomic factors rather than by factors relating to sexual activity. This is important in planning strategies to prevent the condition (Hart, 1992).

Aetiology

Scabies is caused by the mite *Sarcoptes scabiei* (see Figure 14.1). The female of the species burrows into the uppermost layer of the skin and lays eggs, which hatch in about ten days. The female is twice the size of

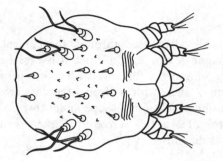

Figure 14.1 Scabies mite.

the male and her mouthparts can just be seen with the naked eye as a black dot. The incubation period is usually 1–3 weeks. During this time the host becomes allergic to the mite's dung, causing the characteristic itching.

Transmission

Transmission occurs through prolonged close physical contact, usually 20 minutes or more. The mite moves slowly, so fleeting contact will not ensure infestation. Sexual contact is ideal for transmission, although the mite can be acquired non-sexually, e.g. between children or in hospitals. Scabies is not usually transmitted by clothes or bedding.

Signs and symptoms

The main symptom is itching. This is often intense and worse at night when burrowing occurs. Lesions can be found in various parts of the body:

- genitals
- in the webs of fingers
- trunk
- wrists and elbows

Burrows can be found on examination and appear as sinuous, scaly red lesions, often 5–15 mm long. As the skin grows the burrows move to the surface. The female mite can be extracted from these. Scratching can alter the appearance of the lesions and can result in:

- eczematous changes
- indurated nodules
- secondary infection

Diagnosis

The condition is usually diagnosed through the clinical history and on examination. The diagnosis can be confirmed if the mite can be extracted. This is achieved by scraping a burrow with a scalpel and placing the collected material on a slide with a drop of potassium hydroxide. The mite can be found using a light microscope under low power.

It is important to offer a full screen for other sexually transmitted infections if scabies is diagnosed.

Treatment

The whole body, including the head, needs to be treated. The following treatments are used:

- 25% benzyl benzoate solution
- 1% gamma benzene hexachloride cream or lotion
- 0.5% malathion

It is useful to alternate treatments for different people in order to prevent resistance. The treatment must be left on for 24 hours and all clothes and bedding should be washed. The itching may persist even after treatment but will gradually disappear. Reapplication of treatment may cause dermatitis.

All sexual contacts must be treated at the same time to prevent reinfection. Contacts who appear asymptomatic must still be treated as they may be incubating the disease.

The use of gamma benzene hexachloride should be avoided in pregnant women as it can appear in the breast milk.

Follow-up

Follow-up of people treated for scabies is important to ensure:

- effectiveness of treatment
- scrutiny of treatment reactions
- contact tracing
- diagnosis and treatment of other sexually transmitted infections.

PEDICULOSIS PUBIS

Epidemiology

This cannot be distinguished from scabies as in England the two conditions are reported together. It has been observed that the incidence of pediculosis pubis appears to be greater among people who (Hart, 1992):

- have multiple sexual partners
- are under 25
- engage in homosexual activity

Aetiology

Pediculosis pubis is caused by a pubic louse called *Phthirus pubis*. This differs from the head and body louse. *Phthirus pubis* is small, 1–2 mm long, and has six legs with clawlike appendages, giving it a crablike appearance, hence it is commonly known as 'crabs'. The claws grasp the pubic hair and other hairy areas. The size of the claws' grip is not suited to the finer hair of the scalp. The louse feeds by injecting saliva into the skin, then sucking the blood.

The female louse lays white oval eggs at the base of the hairs (Figure 14.2). These take about seven days hatch. As the hair grows, the egg can be seen further up the hair shaft. From this it is possible to estimate how recent the infestation is.

Transmission

The lice are transmitted from person to person by physical contact, e.g. sexual contact. They are rarely spread through clothing or bedding as they do not leave the body.

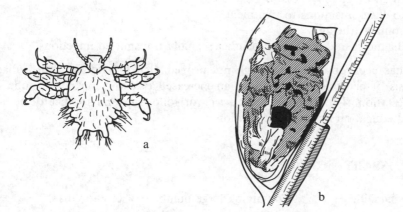

Figure 14.2 Pediculosis pubis louse a) and egg b) not to scale

Signs and symptoms

Sometimes the condition is asymptomatic. The main symptom is irritation of the affected area. The individual may notice the lice and eggs but not realize what they are. The most commonly affected areas are:

- thighs
- perineum
- axillae
- abdomen
- eyelashes
- eyebrows

Diagnosis

This is achieved by clinical examination. Sometimes a magnifying lens can be helpful in locating the lice and eggs. On dark skin it may be difficult to see the lice but the eggs will be visible. The lice can be removed from the skin and examined under a low-power microscope.

Treatment

The treatment is the same as for scabies. All sexual contacts must be treated to prevent reinfection.

Follow-up

Follow-up is important in this condition for the following reasons:

- to check effectiveness of treatment
- to check reactions to treatment
- contact tracing
- diagnosis and treatment of other sexually transmitted infections

It has been observed, although not proved, that individuals with a diagnosis of pediculosis pubis have an increased risk of a further episode of infestation. This reinforces the need for follow-up and for health advice and education about this condition.

GLOSSARY

Eosinophilic	Containing large numbers of eosinophils
Indurated	Lesion with abnormal hardness of the tissue as a result of disease process

REFERENCES

Department of Health (1995) *Statistical Bulletin: Sexually Transmitted Diseases, England 1994.* Bulletin 1995/16.

Hart, G. (1992) Factors associated with Pediculosis pubis and scabies. *Genitourinary Medicine*, **68**(5), 294–6.

Radcliffe, K.W., Daniels, D. and Evans, B.A. (1991) Molluscum contagiosum: a neglected sentinel infection. *International Journal of STD and AIDS*, **2**(6), 416–18.

The patient carrying a parenterally transmitted hepatitis infection

Dinah Gould

OBJECTIVES

1. To describe how the hepatitis A, B, C, D and E viruses are transmitted and diagnosed and their effects on the health of the individual.
2. To list the precautions that should be taken when handling blood or body fluids and explain the rationale underpinning these recommendations.
3. To state the hospital and community health measures taken to control the spread of the hepatitis viruses.

INTRODUCTION

'Hepatitis' is a generic term meaning inflammation of the liver. This can develop for a range of reasons including infiltration by malignant cells (primary tumour, or more commonly metastasis from another site), chemical damage and infection. A number of viruses are able to cause hepatitis, including cytomegalovirus and rubella, but the group of viruses of major concern in the GUM clinic are the hepatitis viruses.

THE HEPATITIS VIRUSES

These are an important cause of both acute and chronic hepatitis. To date, five types of hepatitis virus are commonly discussed in the literature:

- hepatitis A
- hepatitis B

- hepatitis C
- hepatitis D
- hepatitis E

All can give rise to a number of unpleasant symptoms, described and explained below, but only three, hepatitis B, C and D, have the potential to give rise to chronic carrier status. However, all except hepatitis A can result in severe and disabling illness.

SIGNS AND SYMPTOMS

Although only the hepatitis B, C and D viruses are parenterally transmitted and therefore likely to pose a problem with patients attending the GUM clinic, all five types of virus are discussed here because misconceptions about their mode of spread are common, among both the general public and the health care staff who seek to educate them about the risks of transmission and the significance of becoming infected. Additionally, the hepatitis viruses tend to cause infections in young people, who form a high proportion of the typical clientele attending GUM clinics. Patients who discover that they are chronic carriers of hepatitis B or hepatitis C will need particular support and in many cases counselling, because of the possible long-term effects on their health and implications for their sex lives.

The classic signs and symptoms of hepatitis include:

- jaundice (icterus) (a condition characterized by raised levels of plasma biliruben and in more severe cases by yellow skin, sclerae ('whites' of the eyes) and mucosae)
- dark urine
- pale, offensive stools
- pyrexia
- malaise
- tiredness
- anorexia
- nausea
- right-sided abdominal pain

These signs and symptoms are the direct effects of liver damage. The two principal changes in hepatic biochemistry are:

- Disruption of the bile canaliculi, leading to the absorption of conjugated bile into the blood instead of release into the duodenum. Plasma biliruben levels rise and, as bile is needed to emulsify fats, undigested fat is passed in the stools, which become pale and offensive (steatorrhoea).

- Necrosis of the hepatocytes with the release of transferase enzymes (SGOT, SGPT) into the blood. The plasma levels of these hormones become greatly increased, but fall again as the jaundice appears.

Pyrexia occurs as part of the inflammatory response.

The extent to which individuals experience these effects is subject to enormous variation, depending on the severity of their illness and their perception of feeling unwell. Many people have no symptoms at all (subclinical infection) or the symptoms are dismissed because the victim feels vaguely unwell for only a few days and recovers spontaneously without the clinical manifestations of jaundice ever becoming apparent. The pattern and severity of the infection may also depend on the particular hepatitis virus responsible for the infection. Hepatitis C, for example, tends to be particularly damaging, although subclinical infection is also very common.

THE CHARACTERISTICS OF VIRUSES

Viruses are:

1. Minute particles responsible for a wide range of human, animal and plant infections.
2. Obligate parasites, depending on living organisms to provide a host; they do not grow or reproduce outside living cells.

They also have the following characteristics:

3. They lack cellular structure and the characteristics of living organisms.
4. They contain either DNA or RNA, never both.
5. They consist of a protein capsule surrounding a central core of nucleic acid.
6. They are not destroyed by antibiotics; therefore treatment is difficult.
7. 'Enveloped' viruses are surrounded by a lipid and protein capsule with structures permitting them to attach to their hosts.

THE HEPATITIS A VIRUS

The hepatitis A virus (HAV) is an RNA virus. Transmission occurs through the consumption of contaminated food and water. Shellfish like mussels, eaten whole, are an important source because these molluscs feed by filtering particulate matter from seawater. Contaminated material therefore becomes concentrated in them.

Hepatitis A virus infects the bowel as well as the liver, giving rise to a short-term but unpleasant illness. Viraemia (the presence of virus particles in the blood) occurs only transiently and carrier status has never been documented. However, HAV is highly contagious. The infection is particularly likely to be contracted during a holiday abroad, as it is widespread in countries where sanitation is poor and drinking water is subjected to contamination with sewage. Under these circumstances members of the local population will develop immunity through exposure to the virus early in life, but visitors lacking immunity will easily fall victim. It is commonly accepted that an increase in the incidence of HAV is correlated with poor economic circumstances (Cossar, Reid and Fallon, 1990). Outbreaks are common after major disasters such as earthquakes or floods. Cross-infection is possible and has been documented in various types of institution, including schools, prisons and barracks (Kiedzierski, 1991). One of the main reasons that HAV continues to pose a threat to public health is the stability of the virus: it can survive temperatures of 60°C for up to an hour and viable virus particles have been recovered from swimming pools and the sea (Kiedzierski, 1991). The incubation period has been recorded as between two and six weeks, so those returning from a foreign visit may not become ill until some time after their return. Clients may be reassured that recovery from HAV infection will be complete and without long-term effects (Smith, 1993). However, individuals whose lifestyles predispose them to the risks of the parenterally transmitted virus infections may be particularly anxious and will need reassurance that they do not run any risk of becoming chronic carriers.

Diagnosis of HAV infection

Diagnosis of HAV infection is confirmed by the identification of specific antibodies to the virus in the blood.

Treatment of HAV infection

There is no specific treatment.

Public health measures against HAV infection

Effective public health measures in developed countries where an effective system of sanitation exists focus on individuals in particular circumstances:

- Those travelling abroad should be aware of the need to avoid foods eaten raw (fruit, salads). These may have been grown in soil where human excrement has been used as a fertilizer or washed in contaminated water. The need for handwashing should be emphasized and individuals should be aware of the risk of swallowing contaminated water while swimming.

- Travellers may be offered vaccination.
- Those living and working in institutions should be taught the value of frequent and thorough handwashing to prevent cross-infection. This is the single most effective infection control measure (Gould, 1991).
- Anybody in close contact with an individual who has established HAV infection may receive prophylactic immunoglobulin.
- Parents should seek advice before letting previously infected children return to school.
- Those employed in the catering industry and caring professions should not handle food for consumption by others until they are no longer infectious.

THE HEPATITIS B VIRUS

The hepatitis B virus (HBV) is a DNA virus with a long incubation period (3–5 months). It can survive for up to a week in dry plasma (Bond *et al.*, 1983) and is much more infectious than HIV: in situations where an individual has sustained a needlestick injury from a patient carrying both viruses, only evidence of exposure to HBV has later been shown (Gerberding, 1985). Structurally the virus is complex (see Figure 15.1). Information has been derived from studies of its surface antigens. Using recommended WHO terminology, the antigenic structure of HBV is as follows.

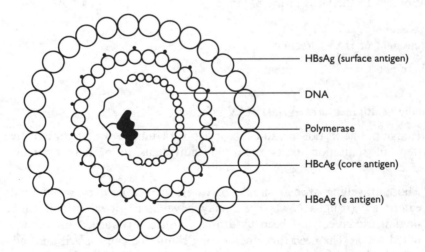

Figure 15.1 The hepatitis B virus.

- Dane particle – the entire virus particle
- HBV – hepatitis B virus
- HBsAg –hepatitis B surface antigen
- HBcAg – hepatitis B core antigen
- HBeAg – the e antigen associated with the core of the virus
- Anti-HBs – antibody to hepatitis B surface antigen
- Anti-HBc – antibody to hepatitis B core antigen
- Anti-HBe – antibody to the e antigen

Infection may follow exposure to blood products and the following body fluids:

- blood
- semen
- vaginal secretion
- saliva

The individual's immune system recognizes the virus and mounts an antibody response. It is thought that this immune response is the factor that damages the liver, leading to the signs and symptoms of hepatitis, because individuals who are immunocompromised generally show evidence of very mild infection. During the immune response, HBV antigens are released and some enter the blood, where they are neutralized. In most cases this leads to resolution of the infection although recovery from acute HBV infection can be prolonged. Unfortunately approximately 5–10% become chronically infected (Hart, 1990). This is probably because the initial immune response is poor and the signs and symptoms of infection do not therefore appear.

Some chronic carriers eventually clear the virus, but a proportion eventually develop cirrhosis or hepatocellular cancer (Main, 1991). Mortality is approximately 1%. In the past, health professionals have tended to be preoccupied with the risks of hepatitis B to themselves, but it is important to keep the risks of parenteral infection in proportion: individuals are most highly infectious during the early, acute stage of the disease, when they are not likely to be attending a GUM clinic. The risks from subclinical infection are, however, considerable: only 30–40% of those infected develop symptoms of acute infection. Transmission occurs sexually (vaginal or anal intercourse), through percutaneous sharps injury, sharing infected needles and by contamination of mucous membranes (mucocutaneous exposure). The risk of infection after percutaneous exposure to the blood of an individual who carries the e antigen, associated with high levels of infectivity, is estimated at about 30% (e.g. 150 out of 500 exposures). The risks associated with mucocutaneous exposure do not appear to have been quantified. Hands may carry minute abrasions not visible to the naked eye, so contamination of apparently intact skin may present a significant risk: it has long been acknowledged that many of those who develop the infection or become carriers cannot recall injury (Denes *et al.*, 1978). The risk of seroconversion depends not only on the nature of the exposure but also on the number of people carrying the virus within the local community and the immunological status of the individual. Despite the high rate of asymptomatic carriage it has long been possible to identify a number of groups who are at high risk (Polakoff, 1986):

- people who inject drugs intravenously;
- homosexual men;
- health professionals;
- immigrants from parts of the world where hepatitis B is endemic: Africa, South East Asia and the Far East;
- people with learning disabilities, especially those in institutional care where hygiene is difficult to control.

Diagnosis of HBV infection

The virus is detected by testing blood for surface antigen (see above). Individuals who have become infected also exhibit raised serum aminotransferase levels. Sometimes biliruben and alkaline phosphatase levels are altered, but these tests are not specific. Blood tests may be used to monitor the resolution and to detect carrier status. For example, resolution of the infection is considered to have taken place when HBsAg and antiHB are no longer detectable. Chronic carriers are those remaining HBsAg positive on at least two occasions six months apart. Infectivity is closely associated with the presence of the e antigen, which indicates that active viral replication is occurring. Attenders are not routinely tested in all GUM clinics. Local policies vary, but in many clinics testing is reserved for those falling into the at-risk groups listed above. Individuals who show no evidence of seroconversion may then be offered vaccination. Those with the e antigen denoting high levels of infectivity will require information to help reduce the risk of spread. They need to understand that they are potentially infectious to sexual partners, so that barrier precautions may be adopted. The risk of infection from blood may be reduced by care with objects likely to become contaminated (never sharing razors, toothbrushes, sewing needles) and by prompt action in the case of blood spillage. In the home the use of bleach (a solution of one part bleach in ten parts water) is recommended.

Treatment of HBV infection

There is no specific treatment for the acute infection, although some individuals are sufficiently ill to require hospital care. Interferon therapy may help clear the virus in 30–40% of chronic carriers (Main, 1991).

Public health measures for HBV infection

HBV infection is notifiable, so all established cases must be reported to the Public Health Laboratory Service so that epidemiological trends can be monitored and the requisite plans for future health need met.

In the community, preventative measures involve:

- screening all blood for transfusion for HBsAg and excluding carriers from donation;
- using small pools of not more than ten donors in the preparation of plasma blood products;
- offering vaccine to those at risk.

In clinical settings, prevention involves the development and implementation of guidelines to prevent transmission from contaminated instruments. A typical infection control policy would advise:

- Care when handling all sharp instruments—they should never be transported in pockets or the hands.
- Needles and syringes should not separated after use.
- Needles used to inject a patient should never be resheathed.
- Prompt disposal of all sharp instruments into a designated container, large enough to hold the complete apparatus without dismantling.
- Disposal of the sealed sharps container when it is no more than two-thirds full. It should be incinerated. Storage before incineration should be in a dry, secure area, free of vermin.
- Prompt action in cases where blood or body fluids are spilt, using sodium dichloroisocyanurate (NaDDC) powder, granules or hypochlorite solution.
- Hepatitis B vaccine is effective prophylactically (Dienstag, Werner and Polk, 1984). If the person has not been immunized, a course of vaccination is suggested.
- Universal precautions (described below). It is not possible to predict whether an individual is carrying a parenterally transmitted viral infection (Havlichek, Greenman and Plaisier, 1991) and, as exposure to blood may occur before testing (Gurevich, 1988), universal precautions must be taken whenever blood or body fluids are handled or if contact is possible (Wilson and Breedon, 1990). This means that risk assessment is of the procedure about to be undertaken, not of the individual patient. In addition, all patients are treated the same, and thus no individual will perceive themself to be stigmatized (Oakley, 1994).

Universal precautions

1. *Gloves* should be worn during all invasive procedures (to protect the patient) and whenever contact with blood or body fluids takes place or

is anticipated (to protect the health professional). They should be changed between patients to prevent cross-infection.

Hands must be washed after gloves have been worn. Latex and PVC may allow the leakage of virus particles (Korniewitz *et al.*, 1989), and allergy may develop to the gloves or the lubricating powder they contain (Van Rijwisjk, 1992).

2. *Aprons* must be worn if clothing is likely to be soiled. Plastic is a more effective barrier against liquid soiling than cotton (Gill and Slater, 1991).

3. *Eye protection* and masks are required only when splashing or aerosols are possible. This is unusual in the GUM clinic.

4. *Sharps* require particular care:
   - Needles should never be resheathed, cut or bent.
   - Needles should never be disconnected from syringes.
   - Sharps containers should comply with British Standard Institute Regulations—be rigid, impermeable, and puncture-proof.
   - Sharps should be placed in a designated container immediately after use.
   - No attempts must ever be made to retrieve items from sharps containers or to empty them.
   - Sharps containers should be discarded when no more than two-thirds full, sealed and stored in a secure, dry place ready for collection. They must be incinerated.

5. *Clinical equipment* must be inspected and decontaminated or replaced as appropriate. Studies have revealed that equipment in immediate patient contact, such as phlebotomy cuffs, may become splashed with blood (Forseter, Joline and Wormser, 1990). This is highly undesirable as HBV can survive for up to a week in dry plasma (Bond *et al.*, 1983).

Venepuncture

This procedure deserves special mention because it is so commonly performed by nurses in the GUM clinic. Some authorities maintain that although, according to universal precautions, gloves should be worn, others point out that manual dexterity may be sacrificed, increasing the risk of infection because needlestick injury becomes a more likely hazard. Two-tier glove wearing, in which gloves are used whenever contact with blood and body fluids is anticipated, but not during venepuncture, is now recommended by many infection control experts (Jenner, 1990).

Immunization

Immunization has been available since the early 1980s. Originally the vaccine was produced from human plasma, but most is now obtained through a recombinant DNA technique which inserts HBsAg into yeast cells. Both vaccines are safe and approximately 90% effective. The duration of immunity has been estimated at 3–5 years. The vaccine should be routinely available to health care professionals and today most Trusts in the UK provide it (Trevelyan, 1991). Side effects are minimal (Finch, 1987). Reasons for the low uptake reported among health professionals include inconvenient appointment times in occupational health departments, pressures of work and misconceptions about the vaccine, especially overlooking the need for boosters (Briggs and Thomas, 1994). Initially it was estimated that only 1–4% of those who had received the standard vaccination, consisting of three injections, failed to respond (Boxall, 1993), but it has since emerged that a higher proportion may be 'slow responders', requiring up to nine injections before seroconversion occurs (Poole, Miller and Fillingham, 1994). This suggests that it is not sufficient to evaluate the successfulness of an immunization campaign merely on uptake: serological testing to determine the effectiveness of the vaccine among recipients is of key importance. Nevertheless, the number of health professionals and members of the public becoming infected with HBV has declined in recent years.

THE HEPATITIS C VIRUS

Once diagnostic tests had become available for hepatitis B it became apparent that a number of postviral cases of hepatitis must be associated with infection by a hitherto unknown agent, initially termed non-A non-B hepatitis. This proved to be an RNA virus subsequently named hepatitis C (Feinstone, Kapitan and Purcell, 1975). The hepatitis C virus (HCV) has an incubation period of about 50 days (Murrell, 1993). It is transmitted primarily via blood and body fluids, although in the USA approximately 10% of those infected appear to have no apparent risk factor. Nevertheless, HCV appears to be most common among intravenous drug abusers and is now thought to occur more frequently in this population than does HIV or HBV in some parts of the USA (Kelen, Green and Purcell, 1992). Sexual transmission is also thought to be possible and asymptomatic carriage is common (Tedder, Gibson and Briggs, 1991). Needlestick injury may lead to seroconversion in health care workers (Polish, Toing and Co, 1993) and has been estimated to place the individual at a 3–10% risk of infection (Mitsui, Inano and Masuka, 1992). Chronic carriage may currently affect as many as 300,000 people in the United Kingdom. The hepatitis C virus appears to be a potentially more damaging infection than HBV. In studies conducted so far, 50% of those infected become chronic carriers and of these 20% develop hepatocellular cancer. Seroconversion may not occur until several months after exposure to the infectious agent.

Diagnosis of HCV infection

Diagnosis of HCV infection is confirmed by the identification of specific antibodies to the virus in the blood. Tests are less sophisticated than for HBV. A positive result indicates that the individual has been exposed to the virus and that the immune system has responded. Tests currently available cannot distinguish between active and old infections or indicate whether or not the individual is infectious.

Treatment of HCV infection

Interferon therapy appears to hold promise for those with chronic HCV infection (Smith, 1993).

Public health measures for HCV infection

The measures detailed above for HBV infection apply. Routine screening of donated blood did not commence until September 1991 in the United Kingdom, but was established earlier in the USA and most other European countries. Vaccination is not yet possible. Opportunities for health promotion are less good than for infection with HBV because blood tests yield less information about the state of the infection and because prophylaxis cannot yet be offered. At present, attenders are not, therefore, routinely tested in GUM clinics.

THE HEPATITIS D VIRUS

The hepatitis D virus (HDV) was first identified in 1977. It is an RNA virus, also known as the 'Delta virus', and has an incubation period of between 30 and 50 days (Murrell, 1993). The hepatitis D virus is described as a 'defective' virus as it is able to cause infection only in the presence of active HBV infection: the two may occur simultaneously or HDV infection may develop in an individual already infected with HBV. Thus transmission is parenteral. It is particularly likely to occur in intravenous drug users and haemophiliacs. Mortality from acute HDV infection is high; 2–20% in outbreaks so far reported. Hepato-cellular cancer appears more likely to develop than with chronic carriage of HBV.

Diagnosis of HDV infection

Infection is diagnosed by detecting the antigen (HDAg) in the blood. Little is known of its prevalence because routine testing is not performed.

Treatment of HDV infection

Interferon therapy may be helpful (Main, 1991).

Public health measures for HDV infection

As transmission can occur only in the presence of active HBV infection, HDV is susceptible to the same preventative strategies.

THE HEPATITIS E VIRUS

The hepatitis E virus (HEV) is a recently discovered hepatitis virus disseminated in the same manner as HAV, by the faecal–oral route. The incubation period appears to be in the region of 50 days (Murrell, 1993). Carrier status has not been reported. The infection has been detected in travellers, chiefly young adults returning to the USA from Asia, Africa and Mexico.

Diagnosis of HEV infection

Diagnosis of HEV infection is confirmed by the identification of specific antibodies to the virus in the blood.

Treatment of HEV infection

There is no specific treatment.

Public health measures for HEV infection

Health education programmes for travellers to affected regions should focus on the preventative strategies discussed above in relation to HAV. Emphasis should be placed on the lack of an effective vaccine and the short-lived nature of natural immunity.

GLOSSARY

Body fluids   Collective term for blood and all blood products, semen, vaginal fluid, saliva, unfixed tissues and organs, urine and faeces (Royal College of Nursing, 1994)

Hepatitis   Inflammation of the liver

Jaundice (icterus)	Condition characterized by raised levels of plasma biliruben and in more severe cases by yellow skin, sclerae ('whites' of the eyes) and mucosae
Parenteral transmission	Delivery of a substance by any route other than via the alimentary tract (today usually taken to mean transmission via blood)
Sharp	Any item able to cut or penetrate skin or mucous membranes (needles, razors, lancets, scalpel blades, microscope slides, ampoules, wires, stitch cutters (Royal College of Nursing, 1994).
Universal precautions	Precautions taken routinely during contact with blood or body fluids: wearing gloves and a plastic apron, decontaminating hands after removing gloves (Wilson and Breedon, 1990)
Viraemia	Presence of virus particles in the blood

REFERENCES

Bond, W.W., Favero, M.F., Peterson, M.J. *et al.* (1983) Inactivation of hepatitis B virus in intermediate to high level disinfectant chemicals. *Journal of Clinical Microbiology*, **18**, 535–38.

Boxall, E.H. (1993) Risks to surgeons and patients from HIV and hepatitis. *British Medical Journal*, **306**, 652–3.

Briggs, M. and Thomas, J. (1994) Obstacles to hepatitis B vaccine uptake by health care staff. *Public Health*, **108**, 137–48.

Cossar, J.H., Reid, D. and Fallon, R. (1990) A cumulative view of studies on travellers—their experiences of illness and the implications of these findings. *Journal of Infection*, **21**, 27–42.

Denes, A.F., Smith, J.L., Maynard, E.E. *et al.* (1978) Hepatitis B infection in physicians. Results of a nationwide seroepidemiological study. *Journal of the American Medical Association*, **239**, 210–11.

Dienstag, J.L., Werner, B.G. and Polk, B.F. (1984) Hepatitis B vaccine in health care personnel: safety, immunogenicity and indicators of efficacy. *Annals of Internal Medicine*, **101**, 34–40.

Feinstone, S.M., Kapitan, A.Z. and Purcell, R.H. (1975) Transmission-associated hepatitis not associated to viral hepatitis A or B. *New England Journal of Medicine*, **292**, 767–70.

Finch, R.G. (1987) Time for action on hepatitis B vaccination. *British Medical Journal*, **294**, 197–8.

Forseter, G., Joline, C. and Wormser, G.P. (1990) Blood contamination of tourniquets used in routine phlebotomy. *American Journal of Infection Control*, **18**, 386–390.

Gerberding, J.L. (1985) Transmission of hepatitis B without transmission of AIDS by accidental needle stick. *New England Journal of Medicine*, **31**, 56–7.

Gill, J. and Slater, J. (1991) Building barriers against infection. *Nursing Times*, **87**(50), 53–4.

Gould, D. (1991) Nurses' hands as vectors of hospital-acquired infection: a review. *Journal of Advanced Nursing*, **16**, 1216–25.

Gurevich, I. (1988) Complications of ICU hospitalisation. Transmissible infections in critical care. *Heart and Lung*, **17**, 331–4.

Hart, S. (1990) Hepatitis B: guidelines for infection conntrol. *Nursing Standard*, **4**(45), 24–7.

Havlichek, D.H., Greenman, E. and Plaisier, K. (1991) High prevalence of historical risk factors for blood-borne infections among in-patients in a community hospital. *American Journal of Infection Control*, **19**, 67–72.

Jenner, E. (1990) Seeking a rationale for glove use. *Nursing Times*, **86**(12), 73–4.

Kelen, G.D., Green, G.B. and Purcell, R.H. (1992) Hepatitis B and hepatitis C in emergency department patients. *New England Journal of Medicine*, **326**, 1399–1404.

Kidzierski, M. (1991) Management of viral hepatitis. *Nursing Standard*, **5**(42), 29–32.

Korniewitz, D.M., Laughton, D., Butz, A. and Larson, E. (1989) Integrity of vinyl and latex procedure gloves. *Nursing Research*, **38**, 144–6.

Main, J. (1991) Therapy of chronic viral hepatitis. *Journal of Hospital Infection*, **18**, (Supplement A), 177–83.

Mitsui, T., Iwano, K. and Masuka, K. (1992) Hepatitis C virus infection in medical personnel after needlestick accident. *Hepatology*, **16**, 1109–14.

Murrell, A. (1993) Unlocking the virus. *Professional Nurse*, **8**(12), 780–3.

Oakley, K. (1994) Making sense of universal precautions. *Nursing Times*, **90**(27), 35–6.

Polakoff, S. (1986) Acute viral hepatitis B: laboratory reports 1980–1984. *British Medical Journal*, **293**, 37–8.

Polish, L.B., Toing, M.J. and Co, R.L. (1993) Risk factors for hepatitis C virus infection among health care personnel in a community hospital. *American Journal of Infection Control*, **21**, 196–200.

Poole, C.J.M., Miller, S. and Fillingham, G. (1994) Immunity to hepatitis B among health care workers performing exposure prone procedures. *British Medical Journal*, **309**, 94–5.

Royal College of Nursing (1994) *Guidelines on Infection Control for Nurses in General Practice*, RCN, London.

Smith, J.P. (1993) Hepatitis C: a major public health problem. *Journal of Advanced Nursing*, **18**(3), 503–6.

Tedder, R.S., Gibson, R.J.C. and Briggs, M. (1991) Hepatitis C virus: evidence for sexual transmission. *British Medical Journal*, **302**, 1299–302.

Trevelyan, J. (1991) Hepatitis B and the law. *Nursing Times*, **87**(9), 52–3.

Van Rijwisjk, L. (1992) Gloves and other rubber-based devices: benefits, problems and guidelnes. *Wounds: A Compendium of Research and Practice*, **4**, 65–73.

Wilson, J. and Breedon, P. (1990) Universal precautions. *Nursing Times*, **86**(37), 67–9.

16	# Human immunodeficiency virus

OBJECTIVES

1. To describe the microbiology of human immunodeficiency virus (HIV) and its effect on the immune system.
2. To state the main modes of transmission of HIV.
3. To explain the stages of HIV infection.
4. To recognize the common opportunistic infections and conditions associated with HIV.
5. To describe the ways in which HIV is diagnosed.
6. To explain the many therapies associated with HIV.
7. To discuss the importance of prevention strategies against HIV.

SUMMARY

This chapter describes the management of individuals with HIV on an outpatient basis in a GUM clinic. A full description of the microbiology of HIV is included and the modes of transmission are discussed. The symptomology of HIV and AIDS is described with details of opportunistic infections and other conditions. The main diagnostic methods are explained and issues around HIV testing are discussed. Rather than listing treatments for each of the opportunistic infections, we present an overview of current antiretroviral therapy and emphasize the importance of prevention.

EPIDEMIOLOGY

Human immunodeficiency virus is a relatively new infection; the first recorded death from AIDS in England occurred in 1985. The number of reported cases of HIV has grown since then to 22,000 in 1994, as a result of both endemic spread and cases imported from abroad (PHLS Communicable Disease Surveillance Centre, 1994). In 1994, 1,343 new cases of asymptomatic HIV were recorded in England – a similar figure to previous years.

Although in the United States and the United Kingdom AIDS was first recognized in homosexual men, it soon became apparent that this disease was not confined to this group. Globally most people now become infected through heterosexual sex; in some countries this has been the case since the start of the epidemic.

HIV and AIDS occur in most countries in the world, with an estimated three million cases of AIDS in total (WHO, 1993). The epidemiology of HIV is discussed fully in Chapter 3.

MICROBIOLOGY

Human immunodeficiency virus is a retrovirus belonging to the lentivirus subfamily. In the late 1970s and early 1980s the incidence and mortality of previously benign opportunistic infections began to rise and acquired immune deficiency syndrome (AIDS) was recognized. It was found to be caused by the retrovirus HIV-1. A variant of this, HIV-2, was isolated later.

Human immunodeficiency virus is icosahedral in shape, has an envelope and is 100–120 nm in diameter. It contains ribonucleic acid (RNA) and an enzyme, reverse transcriptase. This enzyme enables the virus to make a deoxyribonucleic acid (DNA) copy of its own RNA to allow it to integrate into the genetic material of the host cell. Once in control of the host cell, it can instruct it to produce more RNA viruses.

Human immunodeficiency virus possesses outer glycoproteins (gp120) which bind with host receptors (CD4) on particular cells in the body, e.g. T4 helper cells (CD4 lymphocytes), monocytes, macrophages and others. The virus enters these cells by endocytosis (membrane fusion), then sheds its viral coat to release RNA and reverse transcriptase into the cell. Using this enzyme the RNA is copied to DNA then enters the host cell nucleus and integrates with the host DNA. The virus may now become latent until stimulated, a mechanism that is poorly understood. Once reactivated, new viruses are made, then exit the cell by budding and target new cells. The budding process damages the host cell, causing it to die. (See Figure 16.1.)

Human immunodeficiency virus has a devastating effect on the immune system. Not only does it directly affect the T4 helper cells, macrophages and monocytes, but it destroys the efficiency of the entire immune system. The ability of B lymphocytes to produce antibody is affected, as

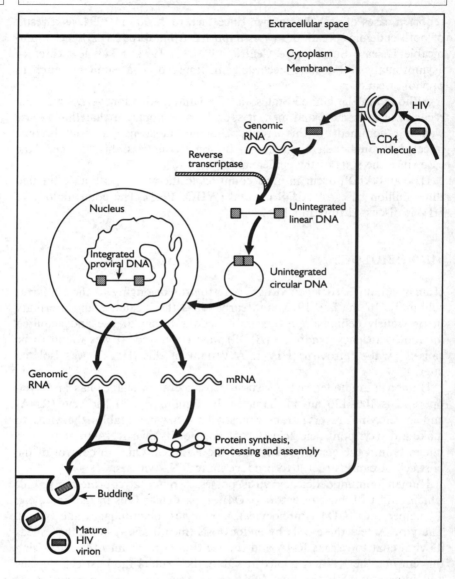

Figure 16.1 The life cycle of HIV.

is the function of CD8 lymphocytes. The body finds it increasingly difficult to destroy neoplastic and virus-infected cells and bacteria.

HIV-2 is closely related to HIV-1 and is currently found in most West
African countries. It is possible that other variants of the virus will be
discovered.

TRANSMISSION

Human immunodeficiency virus is a blood-borne virus and is found in:

- blood
- semen
- vaginal fluid
- breast milk
- cerebrospinal fluid
- saliva
- tears

Human immunodeficiency virus is very fragile and not easily transmitted. The virus will not survive very long outside the body if unprotected by body fluids and is destroyed by heat, drying or detergents. It is transmitted from person to person by:

- sexual contact; exchanging body fluids
- exposure to infected blood or blood products
- vertical transmission from mother to baby

Sexual contact

It is known that certain sexual practices carry a higher risk of HIV transmission than others, e.g. unprotected vaginal and anal intercourse. Oral sex is considered to be lower risk as the concentration of HIV in saliva is relatively low. Any sexual practices resulting in trauma to mucous membranes and exchange of fluids such as semen, vaginal secretions and blood will increase the risk of transmission of HIV.

Exposure to infected blood and blood products

Human immunodeficiency virus can be transmitted by individuals sharing contaminated needles and syringes. Some users of injected drugs may also be more at risk of acquiring HIV through sexual intercourse due to the effects of drugs that may inhibit normal caution and lead to chaotic lifestyles.

Transmission of HIV has also occurred through the administration of contaminated blood transfusions and blood products such as Factor VIII, used in the treatment of haemophilia, before all donor blood was screened for HIV. In countries where facilities are unavailable for testing blood, HIV transmission still occurs this way.

Similarly there is a potential risk of HIV transmission from donor organs. All individuals donating blood or organs should be tested for HIV but if they have acquired a recent infection the test result will remain negative for up to three months. Therefore, a small risk of HIV transmission still remains.

Health care professionals and others exposed to blood and body fluids are at risk of acquiring HIV and other blood-borne infections unless universal precautions are adhered to. Further discussion of these precautions can be found in Chapter 15.

Vertical transmission

There are several ways in which HIV can be transmitted from mother to baby:

- in the uterus
- during delivery
- after delivery, through breast milk

The risk of vertical transmission various significantly according to the stage of the mother's illness. If the mother has recently acquired HIV or has AIDS the risk of transmission is greater because of the increased amount of free virus in the bloodstream at these times. The risk can be reduced by planning pregnancy as far as possible to avoid these times and by avoiding breast feeding. Recent studies have shown that using zidovudine in pregnancy and during birth can significantly lower the transmission rate (Connor et al., 1994).

Other factors

- Different strains of both HIV-1 and HIV-2 may be more virulent than others.
- The presence of other sexually transmitted infections, e.g herpes, may damage the mucus membranes of the vagina or rectum, increasing the likelihood of HIV transmission.
- Individuals are more infectious shortly after infection with HIV and when they become symptomatic. The likelihood of transmission through sexual intercourse is increased at these times.
- Circumcised men are at a greater risk of acquiring HIV than are uncircumcised men.
- The risk of contracting HIV increases with increasing numbers of sexual partners.

SIGNS AND SYMPTOMS

Initial HIV infection is often asymptomatic. Some individuals may experience an acute illness 2–6 weeks after infection, sometimes known as 'seroconversion illness'. This has general manifestations such as malaise, fever, headache and joint pains. In addition some individuals may develop lymphadenopathy.

These are all signs of seroconversion as the body begins to produce antibodies to HIV.

Once seroconversion has occurred, the individual may remain symptom-free for a considerable length of time, it is thought up to 15 years in some cases. During this time, changes in the blood can be monitored e.g. reduction in the number of lymphocytes.

Some individuals develop persistent generalized lymphadenopathy (PGL). This is characterized by lymph node enlargement at two or more extra-inguinal sites for more than three months.

Early symptomatic disease is recognized in individuals with HIV presenting with minor opportunist infections, for example:

- skin conditions like seborrhoeic dermatitis
- oral candidiasis
- hairy leukoplakia on the tongue
- reactivated *Herpes simplex*
- diarrhoea
- fungal infections such as *Tinea cruris*
- malnutrition

AIDS

At this stage opportunistic infections have established clinical illness in a compromised immune system. Commonly, several infections are present at once. A wide variety of infections may be involved, including the following.

Protozoal infections

- *Pneumocystis carinii*, causing pneumonia
- *Toxoplasma gondii*, causing encephalitis and rarely pneumonia and myocarditis
- *Cryptosporidium*
- *Giardia lamblia*
- *Entamoeba histolytica*
- *Isospora*

The last four infections all cause diarrhoea.

Bacterial infections

- *Mycobacterium tuberculosis*

- *Mycobacterium avium-intracellulare*
- *Mycobacterium kansasii/xenopi*

(All the above bacteria can cause pulmonary disease, lymphadenopathy and disseminated disease.)

- *Salmonella typhimurium*, causing diarrhoea and septicaemia
- *Shigella flexneri*, causing enteritis and bacteraemia
- *Legionella*
- *Listeria monocytogenes* can cause meningitis
- *Nocardia* can cause brain, skin and pulmonary abscesses
- pyogenic bacteria, e.g. haemophilus, streptococcus (including pneumo-coccus)

Fungal infections

- *Candida albicans,* affecting the oesophagus
- *Cryptococcus neoformans*, causing meningitis
- *Aspergillus* can cause pneumonia
- *Coccidioides immitis* can cause disseminated disease and meningitis
- *Tinea spp*

Viral infections

- cytomegalovirus can cause ulceration of the gastro-intestinal (GI) tract, pneumonitis and retinochoroiditis which may lead to blindness;
- *Herpes simplex* may cause severe perianal or facial lesions;
- *Herpes zoster*, causing shingles;
- Epstein–Barr virus, causing fever and lymphadenopathy;
- papovaviruses (JC/SV6-40) can cause progressive multifocal leuco-encephalopathy (PML).

In addition to these various infections commonly seen in individuals with HIV, certain malignancies may also arise. Kaposi's sarcoma (KS) was a relatively unusual vascular tumour before the advent of HIV. These aggressive tumours manifest themselves as discoloured patches or nodular lesions on any part of the body. They are often found in the mouth and can be present in the lungs, spleen, liver and GI tract. Kaposi's sarcoma is an AIDS-defining illness, with only a quarter of all patients surviving more than two years.

Undifferentiated lymphomas are also seen in individuals with HIV although not as commonly as KS. These can affect various sites including the GI tract and central nervous system. Invasive cervical cancer is more common in women with HIV disease.

DIAGNOSIS

There are several methods for the detection of HIV.

Serology

Routine screening for HIV is achieved using enzyme-linked immuno-sorbent assay (ELISA). This test measures antibodies to one or more envelope proteins, e.g gp120, and can detect both HIV-1 and HIV-2. Sometimes false positive results occur with this method. To confirm positive tests more specific procedures are used, such as Western blot or immunofluorescent assay (IFA). Western blot involves the identification of individual viral proteins. It is a complicated test and difficult to conduct. Immunofluorescent assay can also detect HIV antibodies but is too time consuming to use as a screening test.

These tests do not give any information about the stage of the disease. In some individuals it can take up to three months for HIV antibodies to be detected in the serum. This is sometimes known as the 'window period'. Therefore testing is advised three months after the individual has been at risk.

Antigen assays

In 60% of individuals with HIV, p24 antigen can be detected, suggesting that active viral replication is taking place (Murray *et al.*,1990). This occurs 2–3 weeks into acute infection and when the individual becomes symptomatic. It is not detected when the virus is latent.

Polymerase chain reaction

This method measures HIV nucleic acid. It is not a general screening test but, as it can detect HIV nucleic acid at a very low level, it can be useful for detection in children.

Culture

This is a complex procedure but can detect even latent virus. It is achieved by noting the appearance of reverse transcriptase and detecting p24 antigen in the medium.

Immunological studies

CD4 lymphocytes are decreased in HIV infection and measurement of these can indicate, though not definitely diagnose, the presence of HIV infection.

Many issues surround the subject of HIV testing. In the United Kingdom it is generally recognized that individuals requesting HIV testing should be counselled about the implications and advantages and disadvantages of consenting to a test. It is a legal requirement, as with all medical procedures, that individuals should have the opportunity to give informed consent before HIV testing is carried out. In GUM clinics pre-test and post-test counselling is generally carried out by health advisers. In some cases nursing and medical staff are also involved.

Pre-test counselling

- A sexual history is taken.
- Risk factors are established and discussed.
- Implications for life insurance and mortgages are discussed.
- Coping strategies are explored.
- Support networks are discussed.
- The meanings and implications of negative, equivocal and positive results are explained.
- The advantages and disadvantages of testing are discussed.
- Confidentiality is assured.

Advantages of HIV testing

- If the test proves positive the individual can be monitored closely and prophylaxis for opportunistic infections initiated.
- It may help women to make decisions about childbearing.
- It is an opportunity for health education, and possible behaviour change.
- Medical decisions may be necessary, in the case of transplant surgery for instance.

Disadvantages of HIV testing

- The psychological effects of a negative or positive result.
- Individuals may become complacent about safer sexual practices if the result is negative.
- Difficulty obtaining mortgages and insurance.

It is essential that all these issues are discussed before testing is carried out.

Post-test counselling

This is important whatever the final result of the HIV test. It is ideal for the the same person, usually a health adviser or a nurse, to perform both the pre-test and post-test counselling so as to provide consistency and continuity.

HIV negative result

To most people this a huge relief. However, in certain circumstances other feelings may be experienced. If the individual has a partner who is HIV positive they may feel guilty about their own result and may need additional support. A further test may be necessary if the window period is a factor and this can be arranged at this visit. Once the negative result is given, there is an ideal opportunity for safer sex issues to be discussed and condoms offered.

Equivocal result

In some ways this is the worst outcome, due to the uncertainty engendered. Often such a result is due to a problem with the testing kit. Occasionally this result is due to seroconversion. The person receiving this result will usually need a great deal of support.

HIV positive result

This is a stressful time for the individuals receiving and giving the result. Every individual reacts in a different way and must be allowed to express their feelings freely. A lot of information is available and needs to be given at this stage but the person may not be able to take it in because of the shock of hearing the result (Firn and Norman, 1995). Follow-up appointments should be encouraged in order for the relevant information to be offered about medical care, partner notification, safer sex and support. Written information is useful as this can be taken away and read at leisure.

TREATMENT

There is no cure for HIV or AIDS at the present time. However, with various forms of intervention many of the opportunistic infections common in HIV disease can be prevented. In addition, anti-viral drugs can help to control the replication of the virus itself and slow down its progress. In GUM clinics, individuals with HIV disease are cared for on an outpatient basis, in principle to keep them as healthy as possible in order to avoid hospital admission. The progression of HIV can be monitored in this way and intervention started when necessary. Opportunistic infections can be treated promptly and preventative measures taken depending on the stage of the illness.

In many GUM clinics certain nursing procedures can be carried out on an outpatient basis. These include blood transfusions, induced sputum for the diagnosis of PCP and inhaled or intravenous pentamidine for the prevention of PCP. Certain procedures and the administration of drugs can be carried out in the patient's home. This is often facilitated by a clinical nurse specialist who will care for patients in the community, liaising closely with the GUM clinic.

It is important for patients to attend as regularly as advised in order for nursing and medical intervention to be successful. There may be reluctance to attend the clinic for various reasons including fear of disclosure of the diagnosis and loss of confidentiality. Also many people with HIV are asymptomatic and regular attendance at the clinic is a constant reminder of HIV and its almost inevitable progression. It is often the nurse who is a constant presence at the clinic and is thus ideally placed to support and advise through these difficult times. Regular clinic attendances can cause disruption and difficulties for life and work as well as psychological problems. Health advising, counselling and psychology services can be accessed through the GUM clinic to provide support for individuals, their partners and families. Other services, such as dietetic, physiotherapy and social work, can also be accessed in this way. If more intensive monitoring or therapy is required the individual will be admitted into hospital as GUM clinics are not usually equipped for such activity.

Monitoring

CD4 lymphocyte counts

There are several ways in which the progression of HIV can be monitored. The most popular method of monitoring until recently has been flow cytometry or CD4 lymphocyte count. As previously discussed, HIV has an affinity for CD4 lymphocytes and measurement of the number of these in the blood can help to monitor the progression of the disease. It is important to bear in mind that CD4 lymphocyte counts vary in people without HIV, thus results of these tests must not be viewed singly but over a period of time and in conjunction with clinical findings. CD4 counts are useful when decisions are made about prophylactic treatments and the introduction of antiretroviral therapies.

Viral load

Recently a new monitoring tool for HIV, viral load, has been hailed as the most useful investigation yet, for two reasons:

- It appears to be the best laboratory marker for disease progression especially in the early stages of the disease (Mellors et al., 1996). It is also thought that, as the CD4 count appears to be a more accurate prognostic marker in the later stages of the disease, these two tests could be used in conjunction with each other (Yerly *et al.*, 1996).

- It appears to be the best marker for predicting the response to antiretroviral therapy (Mellors, 1996).

In summary, viral load testing allows clinicians to identify individuals with HIV who have the greatest likelihood of rapid disease progression, and enables them to monitor accurately the effects of antiretroviral therapies.

Antiretroviral therapy

Antiretroviral therapy is important in the prevention of opportunistic infections and other conditions associated with HIV disease. If the immune system is competent the individual will remain relatively healthy. Once it is compromised it will be open to attack and so monitoring is important in order to initiate prompt diagnosis and treatment.

Initially one antiretroviral drug was used (e.g. zidovudine) but the advantages of using combination therapies have now been demonstrated. Combinations of up to three or four drugs in late disease have been shown to reduce viral replication significantly. These combinations consist of reverse transcriptase inhibitors, e.g. zidovudine, 3TC and a protease inhibitor, e.g. indinavir. As with all drugs, there are problems:

1. Side effects are noted, some very severe.
2. Many drug interactions have been noted – a real issue for individuals who already take a cocktail of drugs for the prevention of various infections.
3. HIV is developing resistance to some of these drugs, which has implications for patient adherence.
4. Combination therapies are very expensive, which has implications for the provision of GU and HIV services.

It has been suggested that the introduction of combination therapies in the treatment of HIV can reduce the amount of virus in the blood to almost undetectable levels and vastly improve the CD4 lymphocyte count. Moreover, it has been implied that total suppression of HIV disease may be achieved (Ho *et al.*, 1995). But this notion does not take into account the fact that, although HIV may be eradicated from the blood, other sites such as the brain may still be infected.

There is no doubt that the introduction of combination therapies and viral load testing can improve the quality of life and prognosis of individuals affected by HIV. However, the degree of improvement is particular to each individual and depends on many co-factors, e.g. tolerance of side effects, compliance, drug interactions. Moreover, the cost of such therapies means that the 90% of people with HIV who live in developing countries are unlikely ever to benefit from these advances.

In addition to the continuing work on treatments for HIV and opportunistic infections, the search for a vaccine for HIV is ongoing.

Alternative and complementary therapies can be of great benefit to people with HIV infection. They are used to reduce stress and to assist in pain control and in sleep problems (Royal College of Nursing HIV Nursing Society, 1994). Examples of popular therapies are aromatherapy, massage and reflexology.

FOLLOW-UP AND PREVENTION

Since the advent of HIV, prevention strategies have been implemented all over the world. This was urgently necessary because no treatment or vaccination against the infection was available. The challenge facing health promotion specialists was the difficult task of changing and maintaining behaviour patterns. In developing countries, where, for example, condoms were unavailable in many areas, the problems were enormous. As HIV spreads further into communities, it is important that health promotion strategies are maintained, both to prevent infection and, among those already infected, to encourage behaviour change. A collaborative approach between natural and medical scientists and local organizations and community groups can present a strong force for the education and support of people against the threat of HIV and AIDS.

In GUM clinics, nurses are in an ideal position to provide sexual health education to individuals using the service. The use of safer sex practices for the prevention of HIV will prevent not only this infection but also the other sexually transmitted infections. Nurses are well placed to discuss individual sexual practices and to offer advice about the type and correct use of condoms for each individual. They must be knowledgeable about the varied lifestyles and sexual practices of people using GUM services and should always remain non-judgemental and impartial in order to win trust. As well as receiving practical advice, many people may benefit from discussing how to negotiate with their partners about possible modification of drug or sexual practices in order to reduce the level of risk.

Human immunodeficiency virus affects not only the individual but the whole family and beyond. Common discussions with nurses include issues such as disclosure of status to partners and families. Family members and friends may know little about HIV and its modes of transmission; nurses can assist in education and advice dealing with these issues. It is recommended that partner notification is encouraged, as for other sexually transmitted infections (Department of Health, 1992), and each individual needs support in their decisions on this issue. The Department of Health recommended that each GUM clinic formulate a partner notification policy and provide training to implement this. The poor uptake of these recommendations was initially thought to be due to lack of patient acceptability (Fenton *et al.*, 1997). Further studies have suggested, however, that patient acceptability is high when partner notification is performed in a skilled and professional manner by trained personnel (Mercey, 1994). It is recognized that partner notification is fraught with difficulties and its effectiveness depends upon the trusting relationship built with patients. The nurse, or more often the health adviser, will use their counselling and supportive skills to enable patients to make informed decisions. Staff training and supervision must be provided in order for partner notification to be effective and acceptable to patients and health care workers alike (Shastd, 1992).

Finally it should be acknowledged that caring for people with HIV can be stressful for the health care professionals involved. Close relationships are formed over long periods of time and the contact with death and dying can be overwhelming. Support and supervision for all staff is important. Clinical supervision for nurses is recommended to assist coping with stressful situations and to allow space for these issues to be discussed (Faugier and Hicken, 1996).

GLOSSARY

Encephalitis	Inflammation of the brain
Glycoproteins	Conjugated proteins containing carbohydrate units
Haemophilia	X-linked recessive blood clotting disorder causing a lifelong tendency to excessive bleeding
Hairy leukoplakia	A thickened white patch on a mucous membrane, usually in the mouth, a precancerous condition
Lymphoma	Cancer of the lymphoid tissue
Myocarditis	Inflammation of the heart muscle
Pneumonitis	Inflammation of the lungs
Seborrhoeic dermatitis	Local inflammation of the skin
Vertical transmission	Transmission of a disease or infection from parent to offspring

REFERENCES

Connor, E.D., Sperling, R.S., Gelber, R., *et al.* (1994) Reduction of maternal–infant transmission of human immunodeficiency virus type 1 with ZDV treatment. *New England Journal of Medicine*, **331**, 1173–80.

Department of Health (1992) *Guidance for Partner Notification for HIV*. PL/CO (92), HMSO, London.

Faugier, J. and Hicken, I. (eds) (1996) *AIDS and HIV – The Nursing Response*, London, Chapman & Hall.

Fenton, K.A., Copas, A., Johnson, A.M. *et al.* (1997) HIV partner notification policy and practice within GUM clinics in England: where are we now? *Genitourinary Medicine*, **73**(1), 49–53.

Firn, S. and Norman I.J., (1995) Psychological and emotional impact of an HIV diagnosis. *Nursing Times*, **91**(8), 37–9.

Ho, D.D., Neumann, A.U., Perelson, A.S. *et al.*, (1995) Rapid turnover of plasma virions and CD4 lymphocytes in HIV1 infection. *Nature*, **373**, 123–6.

Mellors, J.W. (1996) Prognostic value of viral load determinations. Paper presented at Turning the Tide Against HIV: Recent Advances in Combination Antiretroviral Therapy (Official Satellite Symposium), X1th International Conference on AIDS, Vancouver.

Mellors, J.W., Kingsley, L., Gupta, P. *et al.*, (1996) Prognostic value of plasma HIV1 RNA quantification in seropositive adult men. Paper presented at X1th International Conference on AIDS, Vancouver.

Mercey, D. (1994) Clinical audit in genitourinary medicine 'Why, Who, What, How and When?' *Genitourinary Medicine*, **68**(4), 205–6.

Murray, P.R., Drew, W.L., Kobayashi, G.S. and Thompson, J.H. (1990) *Medical Microbiology*, Wolfe, USA.

PHLS Communicable Disease Surveillance Centre (1994) AIDS and HIV infection in the United Kingdom: monthly report. *Communicable Disease Report*, **4**(28), 131–4.

Royal College of Nursing HIV Nursing Society (1994) *AIDS/HIV Infection Nursing Guidelines*, 2nd edn, Royal College of Nursing, London.

The Society of Health Advisers in Sexually Transmitted Diseases (Shastd) (1992) Partner Notification Guidelines, MSF.

WHO (1993) Press release WHO/69 (7 September). World Health Organisation, Geneva.

Yerly, S., Perneger, T., Hirschel, B.L., *et al.*, (1996) HIV viraemia influences survival in HIV-infected patients. Paper presented at X1th International Conference on AIDS, Vancouver.

FURTHER READING

Haak Flaskerud, J. and Ungvarski, P.J. (1995) *HIV/AIDS: A Guide to Nursing Care*, 3rd edn, W.B. Saunders Company, Philadelphia.

Pratt, R. (1995) *HIV and AIDS: A Strategy for Nursing Care*, 4th edn, Edward Arnold, London.

Webb, P. (1994) *Health Promotion and Patient Education: A Professional's Guide*, Chapman & Hall, London.

OBJECTIVES

1. To identify the types of microscopes used in GUM and to explain their use.
2. To describe the Gram staining technique.
3. To explain the process of venepuncture.
4. To describe the processes of male and female genital examination and the types of specimens required to enable diagnosis of sexually transmitted infections.
5. To explain how to obtain an accurate cervical smear.
6. To recognize the different interpretations of cervical smear results and their follow-up recommendations.
7. To describe how colposcopy is performed.

INTRODUCTION

Many of the procedures carried out by nurses in GUM clinics are different from those in other areas. In many ways the nurse is more autonomous in this unique setting and the expanding scope of the role is exhibited in many ways. The procedures commonly performed by nurses in the GUM clinic are:

- microscopy
- venepuncture
- specimen collection
- cervical cytology

Other procedures may be carried out by the medical staff with assistance from the nurse or in some cases by nurse practitioners. These include:

- speculum examination
- bimanual examination
- colposcopy

MICROSCOPY

Historically microscopy in GUM clinics was performed by technicians; however, nurses have now taken on this role in order to develop their expertise and to provide continuity of care for the patient.

Microscopes were first used in 1685. Antony van Leeuwenhoek was the first to observe microorganisms with a simple microscope. Since then the field of microbiology has expanded enormously, with many types of bacteria identified and studied. In the 1890s new staining techniques developed by Paul Ehrlich became available to help scientists observe these organisms.

Many types of microscopes are now available for use but in GUM clinics two types of microscopy are commonly used: light microscopy and dark-field microscopy.

Light microscopy

This microscope has two lenses, the ocular lens in the eyepiece and a second lens in the objective near the specimen. A light source passes through the specimen into the eye of the observer. This type of microscope can magnify 40 to 1200 times. The magnification is calculated by multiplying the magnifying power of the ocular lens, which is usually $\times 10$, by the power of the objective lens, this being $\times 10$, $\times 40$ or $\times 100$.

Degrees of magnification

- With the low-power objective the magnification is usually $\times 100$ (10×10); this can be used for locating the specimen on the slide.
- With the dry lens, larger microorganisms such as protozoa can be viewed, the magnification being $\times 400$ (10×40).
- The oil-immersion objective is $\times 100$, thus, with the $\times 10$ ocular lens, a magnification of $\times 1000$ can be achieved. Bacteria can be studied at this magnification.

In order to view the specimen clearly with the oil-immersion lens a drop of immersion oil must be used between the objective lens and the slide; this reduces the scattering of the light. The additional lighting needed at this higher magnification is achieved by the condenser, which adjusts the amount of light and shapes the cone of light entering the objective.

Resolving power

This enables a specimen to be viewed clearly and in detail. It is the ability of the lens to distinguish between two points at a particular distance. This depends on the light source wavelength and the numerical aperture. The standard resolving power is 0.2 μm with the maximum numerical aperture and an oil-immersion lens. This means that two objects (such as bacteria) can be viewed separately if there is a space of 0.2 μm between them (Burton, 1992).

Staining techniques are used in conjunction with this type of microscopy to distinguish between different microorganisms. These are discussed further in this chapter.

Dark-field microscopy

Light microscopes can be converted into dark-field ones by changing the lens. In this type of microscopy the light source originates from the side, so the light reaching the objective is that which is reflected from the specimen. This enables the bacteria studied to appear bright against a dark background. The magnification is × 1000. In GUM clinics this technique is used to search for *Treponema pallidum* and often *Trichomonas vaginalis* in their live state.

In the GU setting it is not necessary to use more powerful microscopes such as transmission electron microscopes or scanning electron microscopes, which can magnify between 10,000 and 200,000 times. Fluorescent microscopes are used in some laboratories to identify *Chlamydia trachomatis*.

Gram staining

In GUM clinics one main staining technique is used to examine bacteria contained in a dried specimen. This particular technique was developed by Hans Gram in 1884, hence it is named the 'Gram stain'. It enables the observer to determine bacterial shape and to differentiate between 'Gram-positive' and 'Gram-negative' types of bacterial cell wall. The Gram-positive bacteria possess layers of peptidoglycan with teichoic acid in their cell wall and stain blue. The Gram-negative bacteria have a thin layer of peptidoglycan covered with lipids and stain red.

Gram staining process (Burton, 1992)

1. The slide is dried over a flame then flooded with crystal violet for one minute.
2. The slide is rinsed with water, then flooded with Gram's iodine and left for one minute.

3. The slide is rinsed with water again and then acetone is used to deco-
   lourize it for 20 seconds.
4. The slide is then flooded with safranin for a further one minute.
5. It is then rinsed with water and dried over a flame. The slide can then
   be examined under the light microscope with immersion oil. The
   Gram-positive bacteria appear blue and the Gram-negative red.

In GUM clinics the most important bacteria to identify by this method
are *Neisseria gonorrhoeae*, which appear as Gram-negative intracellular
diplococci. A culture plate is inoculated in addition to the microscopy as
a confirmation of diagnosis.

Wet preparation

Trichomonas vaginalis are examined while they are still alive; they cannot
be seen once dried and stained. A specimen of vaginal fluid is obtained
and placed in a drop of saline on a slide. A cover slip is placed on top.
This specimen can now be viewed under either the dark-field or low-
power light microscope, where the live organisms can be seen.
   Treponema pallidum is also viewed live under the microscope. In this
case a specimen of serous fluid from a suspect lesion is placed on a slide
with a cover slip on top. This is viewed under the dark-field microscope,
the organisms appearing silver against the dark background.

VENEPUNCTURE

Venepuncture is a skill demonstrated by most nurses in GUM clinics.
In many other departments this may not be the case and the medical staff
or phlebotomists will carry out this procedure.This skill is used with
almost every patient, so the nurse must quickly become proficient and
confident.
   Venepuncture can be the focus for patient anxiety, therefore, as with
any other clinical procedure, it is important to explain it thoroughly. It is
also important to explain the purpose of obtaining the blood sample.
   Some individuals, if they have had a lot of blood tests, may suggest a
suitable vein and this should be considered. Some individuals have
difficult veins, particularly if they have been used for injecting drugs; in
such cases it may take some time to obtain an adequate blood sample
and it may also be painful.
   There are different types of veins (see Figure 17.1), some more suitable
for venepuncture than others (Thorpe, 1991):

● Large veins – prominent and easy to puncture.
● Deep veins – these may not be immediately apparent, requiring palpation to locate them.

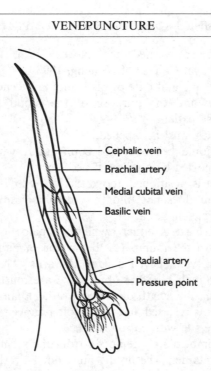

Figure 17.1 The veins and arteries in the arm.

- Thready veins – these can collapse if the blood is taken too quickly.
- Superficial veins – tiny and not suitable for venepuncture.
- Floating veins – these may be large but move when one is trying to puncture them, so they need to be anchored below the puncture site.
- Thrombosed veins – hard and often unusable for venepuncture.

There are several ways is which venepuncture can be performed. Traditionally a needle and syringe were used – and continue to be in some areas. Vacuumed systems have become popular, mainly due to the increased safety for the phlebotomist. Both methods are described here.

Using a needle and syringe

1. All the equipment must be at hand. The essentials are:

   - tourniquet
   - needles
   - syringe
   - cotton wool
   - plaster
   - specimen bottles
   - gloves

2. Hands should be washed and gloves worn, following universal precautions (Royal College of Nursing, 1993).
3. The patient's name and date of birth should be checked.
4. The procedure and the purpose of the blood samples should be explained to the patient.
5. Specimen bottles must be labelled.
6. The patient should be positioned comfortably with the arm straightened and supported by a pillow if necessary.
7. The tourniquet is positioned above the elbow and tightened, ensuring that the patient does not find this too uncomfortable. It may also help if the patient makes a fist.
8. Once a vein is located, either by sight or palpation, it helps to fix it by pressing with the thumb just below the puncture site. The needle is slid into the vein, bevelled edge upwards. The plunger is pulled slowly until enough blood is obtained. Care must be taken to guide the needle along the length of the vein rather than through it.
9. The tourniquet is released and the needle removed. Pressure is applied to the puncture site with cotton wool.
10. The needle is immediately removed from the syringe and disposed of in a sharps container. The needle must not be resheathed. The blood is decanted into the specimen bottles.
11. A plaster is applied to the puncture site, taking care that the patient is not allergic to these. Blood can be taken from the back of the hand if there are no available veins in the arms. This is done in a similar way but a smaller needle may be necessary.

Using an evacuated system

This method enables the blood to be collected straight into the specimen bottle under vacuum. The double-ended needle is screwed into a plastic cylinder and once it is in the vein the specimen bottles are slotted into the cylinder, the rubber cap is punctured by the internal needle and the blood sucked into the bottle. Once all the specimens have been taken, the needle and holder are withdrawn.

This system has safety advantages over the needle and syringe as it is a closed system. The vacuum ensures that there is no risk of spillage and the blood flows straight into the bottle. This eliminates the decanting process required when using a syringe and needle. It is quicker and more convenient, especially when large amounts of blood are required. It is also more cost effective.

The procedure for venepuncture is the same for this system although it may take some practice if the user is used to the needle and syringe method. The needle is discarded after use in the same way. There is some debate about the use of the plastic cylinders for more than one patient.

The manufacturer's instructions and local policies should be followed in this matter. The specimen bottles can also be filled using a syringe and needle if necessary.

The system does have some disadvantages:

- If the user is inexperienced the veins can be traumatized.
- It may be difficult to feel when the needle is in the vein.
- Veins may collapse more easily with this system.

It does appear that the advantages of the evacuated system outweigh the disadvantages, and many hospitals have moved towards this method of blood sampling.

If venepuncture is very difficult to perform on particular patients a fine butterfly needle can be used in smaller veins.

Needlestick injury

Even if the procedure is carried out carefully, there is always a risk of needlestick injuries when performing venepuncture. The use of gloves may help prevent contamination by blood spillage or splashing. If a needle-stick injury is sustained the following action should be taken:

1. The site should be washed with soap and water and encouraged to bleed. It is then covered with a waterproof dressing.
2. The person in charge should be informed and will complete an accident form.
3. A blood sample is taken from the recipient for hepatitis B testing.
4. A blood sample can be taken from the donor if known and, with their consent, tested for hepatitis B.
5. The recipient should seek advice as soon as possible from the GUM consultant or occupational health department about HIV and post-exposure prophylaxis.

All health care staff need to ensure they are vaccinated against hepatitis B and their antibody level should be regularly checked. This will provide protection against hepatitis B in the event of a needlestick injury.

SEXUAL HISTORY TAKING

History taking is a vital part of the management of sexually transmitted infections. It is essential for rapid and accurate diagnosis and gives an indication as to which particular investigations are required. On the first visit to a GUM clinic the sexual history is obtained by the doctor but on subsequent visits this is often the nurse's role. Good history taking requires excellent communication skills as many patients may be reluctant to answer questions about their sex life. They must be reassured of confidentiality, and skilled questioning is necessary to obtain truthful, relevant information. The art of good sexual history taking is learned through practice and observation of others.

FEMALE EXAMINATION

On the first visit to a GUM clinic, female patients should always be examined by a doctor as recommended in the Monks Report (Department of Health, 1988). In the United Kingdom at present it is accepted practice for the medical staff to make the diagnosis and advise on the management of the patient. A nurse practitioner network is slowly developing and once established could be introduced to the field as appropriate. The doctor is usually assisted by a nurse during the examination. On subsequent visits it may be the nurse who performs an examination alone, provided they are competent and confident.

Many women are very nervous at the prospect of having an internal examination so it is important that the atmosphere is as relaxed as possible. All preparation should be completed before the examination; this includes correctly labelling the specimen bottles and culture plates. The following should also be considered:

1. The procedure should be explained fully to the patient. This is often done by the nurse but it may be useful to repeat it even if already explained once by the doctor. Sometimes it helps to show the patient the speculum but only if she wishes.
2. Male examiners should always have a female chaperone. Some women may not want to be examined by a male doctor. It is important when women ask for an appointment at the clinic that there is a choice of male or female staff.
3. The patient should be positioned on the examination couch as comfortably as possible and covered if she prefers. The lithotomy position is usually best (Figure 17.2).

Nurses and other health care professionals performing examinations should follow universal precautions (Royal College of Nursing, 1993) – see Chapter 15.

It is important that the entire genital area is examined systematically, the external genital area first. The examiner needs to be alert for the following:

- parasitic infestation in the pubic area
- warts
- ulcers

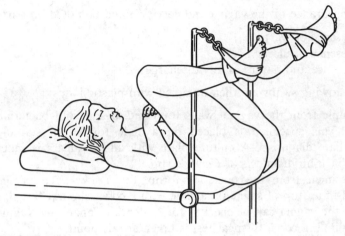

Figure 17.2 The lithotomy position.

- cysts
- swelling or redness
- swelling of inguinal nodes
- any obvious discharge

In addition the size and symmetry of the lower abdomen are observed and any abnormalities like scars, rashes or lesions are noted. The breasts may also be examined.

Once the external examination is complete, the speculum examination is commenced. There are two main types of speculum – Cusco and Sim's. The Cusco speculum is the instrument of choice in GUM clinics as it is easier to view the cervix and more comfortable for the patient. The following considerations should be taken account of:

- Make sure the correct size of speculum is used. For example, if the woman has never had penetrative vaginal intercourse a virginal or small speculum should be used.
- Warm the speculum with water.
- Do not use any other lubrication besides water as this may interfere with the specimens, particularly in cervical cytology.

The speculum should be inserted obliquely, taking care not to pull the pubic hair, pinch the labia or catch folds of the vaginal wall in the blades. Once inside the vagina the speculum is gently rotated so that the blades are horizontal. It can now be opened and secured in position by tightening the screw. The cervix should be fully in view for thorough inspection, and appropriate specimens may be taken. It is important to inform the patient of each stage of the procedure.

The appearance of the vagina and cervix should be noted, in particular:

- the presence of warts
- the presence of ulcers
- the presence and nature of any discharge

The following swabs are then obtained with plastic loops:

1. A sample from the vaginal walls for *Candida* spp. and bacterial vaginosis. This specimen is placed on a slide for Gram staining and immediate diagnosis. A culture plate with added sugars is inoculated for a back-up diagnosis of *Candida* spp.
2. A specimen from the posterior fornix for *Trichomonas vaginalis* is placed in a drop of saline on a slide with a cover slip. At this stage the pH of the vagina can be checked for evidence of anaerobic vaginosis.
3. If required, a cervical smear test is taken at this point.
4. The cervix can then be cleaned with cotton wool to remove excess vaginal fluid. It is debated whether this is useful but it can assist the microscopist as cervical matter can be more easily observed without vaginal contamination.
5. A sample taken from the cervical os for *Neisseria gonorrhoeae* and placed on a slide for Gram staining for immediate diagnosis and culture. The culture plate may contain antibiotics to determine the sensitivity of the bacteria if present.
6. A sample taken from the cervical os for the identification of *Chlamydia trachomatis*. This is processed in the laboratory; immediate detection is not possible in most GUM clinics at present.
7. A general swab for microscopy, culture and sensitivity can be taken here to identify any bacterial infections other than sexually transmitted infections.
8. If indicated, a viral culture for herpes is taken and sent to the laboratory for processing.
9. If indicated, a sample of serum for dark-ground examination is taken by scraping a cover slip across the lesion and mixing serum with normal saline. This can be viewed immediately. When all the specimens have been obtained, the speculum can be withdrawn, slowly bringing the blades closer together.

The last specimen is obtained from 1 cm into the urethra to eliminate gonorrhoea. It is placed on a slide for Gram staining and culture. If gonorrhoea is suspected, a rectal swab is taken (see the section below on rectal examination).

Throat swabs

If gonorrhoea is suspected, a throat swab should be obtained, even if the patient denies having oral sex. The patient is seated with their head tilted backwards and mouth wide open. The tongue is depressed and the swab is taken from the back of the throat and tonsils and directly applied to the culture plate or transport medium.

It is essential that all specimens are carefully treated and preserved, especially if they are transported to the laboratory. Gonococcal samples require special handling. The inoculated culture plates must be immediately placed in anaerobic conditions, incubated at 36°C and transported to the laboratory as quickly as possible.

Bimanual examination

A bimanual examination is the final investigation and is usually carried out by the doctor, although some nurses now perform this procedure. It is an important part of the examination as it is valuable in detecting any abnormal masses in the pelvic region and also pelvic inflammatory disease. Bimanual examination alone cannot be relied on to detect ovarian cancer, so other investigations such as ultrasound scanning are advised.

Bimanual examination is an invasive procedure and should be performed sensitively with a full explanation. Nurses undertaking this require expertise and should receive appropriate training. As stated in the United Kingdom Central Council's *Code of Professional Conduct* (1992), a procedure must not be undertaken unless the nurse is competent to do so and it is the responsibility of the nurse to inform their manager if they have not received appropriate training.

The Royal College of Nursing (1995) advises that bimanual examination is used to assess women who are symptomatic and when clinically indicated.

Other investigations may be necessary and include obtaining midstream urine samples if urinary symptoms are evident, and pregnancy testing if indicated. Patients may be referred to other departments, e.g. ultrasound, gynaecology.

MALE EXAMINATION

On the first visit to a GUM clinic the individual should be examined by a doctor. On subsequent visits the nurse may assess the patient and is often more involved in the examination of male patients than with female patients.

The male genitalia are thoroughly examined with the prepuce retracted. The pubic hair and perianal area should not be ignored. The examiner should be alert to:

- warts
- ulcers
- redness
- swelling, including lymph nodes
- pubic lice and other parasites
- penile or anal discharge

In order for a diagnosis to be made, swabs must be obtained from inside the urethra. This is most effective if the patient has not passed urine for at least two hours and is usually done by passing a plastic loop up to 2cm into the urethra and gently scraping the mucosa. Platinum loops were used for this purpose for many years and have been shown to be the most effective way of collecting urethral specimens. However, this method was most uncomfortable; plastic loops are the most effective alternative (Tang *et al.*, 1992). Several specimens are taken:

1. A urethral specimen for the identification of *Neisseria gonorrhoeae* and NSU is placed on a slide for Gram staining and immediate diagnosis. A culture is also taken for back-up of the microscopy.
2. A urethral specimen for *Chlamydia trachomatis*.
3. If indicated, a swab from the subpreputial area for *Candida albicans*, for immediate diagnosis and culture.
4. If indicated, a urethral swab for *Trichomonas vaginalis*, for immediate examination.
5. If indicated, a viral culture for herpes from sore or ulcerated areas.
6. If indicated, a specimen of serum from an ulcer for a dark-ground preparation to look for *Treponema pallidum*.
7. A specimen for microscopy, sensitivity and culture may be taken if another bacterial infection is suspected.
8. Swabs from the rectum may be taken for gonorrhoea if any anal discharge or soreness is evident (see the section below on rectal examination). A throat swab may also be useful for detection of gonorrhoea.

Once all the urethral tests have been obtained, a urine sample should be collected. This is the two-glass urine test. The patient is asked to pass about 60 ml of urine into one glass and the remainder into a second. Firstly urinalysis can be performed to check for protein, blood or glucose. If the urine is cloudy, 5–10% acetic acid can be added to clear any phosphates; if it remains cloudy and the first glass contains threads and specks, an anterior urethritis may be present, which can be confirmed after the microscopy result is obtained. If there are specks and threads in both glasses, a posterior urethritis or cystitis may be present.

RECTAL EXAMINATION

Rectal examination is performed if rectal symptoms are present and is advisable if the individual, whether male or female, has anal sex. If the nurse is to perform rectal examination, training must be given and the nurse must feel confident about the procedure.

The patient lies in the lateral position or, if a woman, can be examined in the lithotomy position. A proctoscope is lubricated and gently inserted into the anus. Once the introducer is removed, the rectal mucosa can be examined for any erythema, pus, lesions or warts. Swabs can then be obtained as appropriate for gonorrhoea, herpes or microscopy, culture and sensitivity. The proctoscope should be withdrawn carefully and excess lubricating jelly wiped away. If the patient is not complaining of any rectal symptoms, a blind rectal swab can be taken.

The patient can also be referred to other departments if required, e.g. ultrasound, urology.

CERVICAL CYTOLOGY

The concept of cervical cytology was presented in the 1920s by Dr Papanicolaou, who with his colleagues developed a stain that allowed changes due to inflammation or neoplasia to be identified from a smear. This smear can be from any part of the body but cervical smears in particular are discussed in this chapter.

In GUM clinics, cervical cytology is performed when appropriate and many clinics also specialize in colposcopy; thus minor abnormalities of the cervix can be investigated, diagnosed and treated without referral to another department.

Many risk factors have been associated with abnormal cervical cytology including:

- demographic considerations
- low social class
- low age of first sexual intercourse (Farlow, 1993)
- multiple sexual partners
- smoking (Barton *et al.*, 1988)
- human papillomaviruses, especially types 16 and 18
- sperm (celibate nuns rarely develop cervical cancer)
- immunosuppression
- mineral and vitamin deficiencies (Held, 1995)

It has been suggested that people attending GUM clinics may have a high number of these risk factors and recent research has demonstrated that this population also has an increased prevalence of minor cervical smear abnormalities (Young and Malet, 1993). Taking this into consideration, guidelines for cervical screening in GUM include the following (Moss and Hicks, 1994):

- There is a role for GUM clinics in the cervical screening of women who are not entered into the national recall system or who have not had regular screening.
- Follow-up should be locally agreed on the basis of national recommendations.

Screening programmes

In the United Kingdom a cervical screening programme and computerized recall system exist in order to prevent as many cases of cervical cancer as possible. There were 3,768 new cases of invasive cervical cancer in England and Wales in 1991 and in 1994, 1369 women died of this condition. For those women whose condition was diagnosed and treated at an early stage the five-year survival rate was around 90% (NHS Cervical Screening Programme, 1996). A reduction in the number of cases of invasive cervical cancer by at least 20% by the year 2000 is one of the main government targets for health (Department of Health, 1992).

Taking the cervical smear

In GUM clinics the nurse often performs the cervical smear and must be competent and confident in order for the procedure to be performed accurately. For some women this procedure is distressing, especially after a previous bad experience. It is very important to take this into consideration and to make sure the procedure is as comfortable as possible. The first experience of this type of examination may determine whether a woman will return for regular smears. Therefore it is important to conduct the procedure sensitively and gently. It is essential to make clear to the patient that she is having a cervical smear test. In GUM clinics many other tests are taken and this can lead to confusion. It should also be explained how the result is obtained.

The Royal College of Nursing (1996) has issued guidelines for good practice for nurses performing cervical cytology. It is important for the nurse to be competent in the following areas:

- preparation of the equipment and environment;
- assessment of the patient, including history taking and completing the smear form;
- procedure, i.e. visualization and assessment of the cervix, taking an adequate smear and considering the comfort of the patient;

- choosing the appropriate speculum;
- choosing the appropriate spatula.

The traditional device for taking cervical smears is the Ayres spatula. It is ideal for reaching the transformation zone, which may be inside the cervical os. A cytobrush may be used in conjunction with the spatula to ensure the transformation zone has been reached.

1. The speculum can be warmed with water before insertion. The appropriate size speculum is inserted into the vagina as before and positioned to enable a full view of the cervix. Visualization of the cervix can sometimes be difficult. If complete visualization is not possible it is unlikely that an adequate smear will be obtained.
2. Using the bi-lobed end the smear spatula is inserted into the cervical os and turned through 360°, ensuring that the scrape spans the squamocolumnar junction at all points. The cervix is not cleaned or wiped until the smear has been taken.
3. Cervical material is then smeared on to a slide using longitudinal strokes to avoid damaging the cells. The slide is labelled with the clinic number and the client's date of birth.
4. Another sample from the cervical os taken with a cytobrush may be required if the transformation zone is difficult to visualize; this is applied to the slide with a rolling motion.
5. The slide is immediately place in a container with fixative and sent for histological examination. It is suggested that smears should optimally contain:

   - metaplastic cells
   - endocervical cells
   - squamous cells
   - endocervical mucus

A combination of squamous cells and two of the other components constitutes an adequate smear (Austoker, 1994).

Sometimes the cervix may bleed slightly after the smear has been taken, so in order to avoid undue concern the woman should be warned this may happen. It is safe to perform cervical cytology during pregnancy. Once the smear has been examined by a cytologist, a report is written. This contains three sections:

1. Description of the cells

If normal the report may say no abnormal cells seen and suggest a recall date. If abnormalities are detected they may be reported in several ways:

- dyskaryosis due to abnormal changes in the cells, which can be mild, moderate or severe;

- koilocytosis appearing as perinuclear vacuolation of cells due to wart virus infection;
- malignant cells when invasive malignancy is identified.

2. Interpretation of results

At this stage familiar CIN (cervical intraepithelial neoplasia) classification is used. This is the cytologist's impression of the smear pattern and is reported as follows:

- CIN1 mild dyskaryosis
- CIN2 moderate dyskaryosis
- CIN3 severe dyskaryosis to carcinoma *in situ*

Sometimes the cytologist will have difficulty examining the smear and it may be reported as unsuitable for screening. Evidence of inflammation may mean that the smear will need repeating and will be reported as such. In GUM clinics, if an infection is suspected it is worth delaying cervical screening until infection has been excluded or treated (Robinson *et al.*, 1992).

3. Action

This is the advice for follow-up and recall. Recent guidelines (Duncan, 1992) have set a national protocol for the management of cervical screening in response to the increasing rates of cervical cancer, especially in young women. These are based on the concept that CIN can be viewed as a continuum from mild to severe. Some idea of the rate of progression of abnormalities is necessary. Unfortunately this is difficult to predict in the lower-grade abnormalities. Many of these will regress spontaneously, some will persist and others will progress. Acknowledging these difficulties, these guidelines recommend that:

- CIN2 and CIN3 should be treated.
- CIN1 may be treated or closely monitored.
- Colposcopy should be recommended for a moderately or severely dyskaryotic smear.
- Smears showing borderline nuclear or mildly dyskaryotic changes should be repeated in six months' time and then colposcopy offered if the results are still abnormal.
- Following an abnormal smear, there should be two consecutive negative smears six months apart before smears are allowed to return to the normal three-yearly recall.
- Following treatment a smear should be taken after six months, then if normal, after 12 months.
- If HPV is found on a smear, referral to GUM should be considered.

In addition the guidelines suggest that all women should be given detailed written and verbal information at all stages of the cervical screening and colposcopy process.

Practitioners involved in taking cervical smears are responsible for informing women of their results and ensuring that appropriate follow-up is carried out (Pike and Chamberlain, 1992). In some cases women may not want their GP informed and will not be on the national computerized recall system, therefore it is the responsibility of the GUM clinic to manage an effective recall system (Moss and Hicks, 1994).

COLPOSCOPY

Colposcopy is the observation of the cervix with binocular magnification. In 1925 Hinselmann claimed that malignancies of the cervix occurred as minute ulcers or tumours which could be seen with appropriate magnification and illumination. He designed a colposcope and eventually his work was recognized as significant in the study of cervical cancer. It was not until the 1970s that colposcopy became recognized as a valuable technique in the United Kingdom.

The colposcope can be very useful in GUM for the assessment of lesions on the vulva, anus and penis as well as on the cervix. The colposcopist must be adequately trained and confident, and national guidelines for colposcopy should be followed (Moss and Hicks, 1994).

Genitourinary medicine clinics have an important part to play in reaching government targets to reduce the incidence of cervical cancer, and many nurses within the speciality are making a valuable contribution towards this. Nurses are well aware of the need for good communication with patients, especially with those who are anxious about certain procedures. This certainly includes colposcopy and nurses can do much to allay some fears by explaining the procedure, developing written information and setting up support groups. In addition some nurses have trained as colposcopists and are directly involved in the treatment of such patients.

For patients attending a GUM clinic, continuity of care is maintained if colposcopy is available within the clinic. This may lessen the rate of failure to attend. It is still important, however, that close links are kept with gynaecological colleagues.

Women referred for colposcopy from other sources such as GP practices may have anxieties about confidentiality. It is important to discuss this with each individual and to obtain their consent to provide additional information to the referral source. For example it may be acceptable to the individual for details of the actual colposcopy to be disclosed to their GP but they may prefer that information about sexually transmitted infections remains confidential.

The indications for colposcopy are discussed above in the section on cervical cytology.

Procedure

A sexual history is taken from the patient, including information about their menstrual cycle, pregnancies, contraception, smoking and previous cervical treatment, all of which can affect the appearance of the cervix. It is important at this stage that the patient is given a full explanation of the procedure and time to ask questions.

The patient must be in the lithotomy position as if she were having a cervical smear. The nurse's role is vital here to assist the patient, provide support and help to maintain dignity. In the GU setting a basic screen for sexually transmitted infections is often carried out at this point. The presence of an infection such as chlamydia can often cause inflammatory appearances on cervical smears.

The colposcope is then positioned and focused. A clear view of the whole of the cervix is essential. It is important to explain each stage of the procedure to the patient.

1. Aceto-white test

Dilute acetic acid (5%) is applied to the cervix. This may sting slightly. Areas containing the human papillomavirus will show up with varying degrees of whiteness.

2. Schiller's test

This is used by some colposcopists and may be useful in outlining the extent of the abnormal area. Lugol's iodine is applied to the cervix. This reacts with the glycogen present in healthy squamous cells and stains dark brown. Abnormal areas producing less glycogen will appear lighter and can be more easily identified.

Once the area of abnormality is defined, small biopsies are taken for histological examination. Some patients may not feel this but others may experience a sensation similar to period pain. The bleeding is usually controlled using a silver nitrate stick or Monsel's solution. The patient must be warned that they may experience bleeding or a brown discharge for a few days and that sexual intercourse should be avoided until the discharge stops. A follow-up appointment is made for discussion of results.

A decision is made about further treatment when the biopsy result is available. Treatment such as cold coagulation or cryotherapy can be performed in the GU clinic by staff who have been trained in these procedures. More radical treatments, such as laser treatment, loop diathermy or cone biopsy, may need to be carried out in a better equipped location, often by a gynaecologist.

GLOSSARY

Bimanual examination   Performed using both hands, one hand placed on the abdomen and one or two fingers in the vagina

Cone biopsy   The removal of a cone-shaped segment of tissue from the neck of the womb to provide material for positive microscopic diagnosis

Cryotherapy   The use of low temperatures in medical treatment; −20°C is good for destroying unwanted tissue

Dyskaryosis   A visible abnormality in the nuclei of cells that appear otherwise normal

Lithotomy position   The individual lies on his or her back with the knees up and thighs spread wide, and the feet and thighs usually supported in slings

Venepuncture   Entry into a vein, usually with a hollow needle to gain access to the bloodstream for the purpose of obtaining a sample of blood or giving an injection directly into it.

REFERENCES

Austoker, J. (1994) Screening for cervical cancer. *British Medical Journal*, **309**, 241–8.

Barton, S.E., Maddox, P.H., Jenkins, D. *et al.* (1988) Effect of cigarette smoking on cervical epithelial immunity: a mechanism for neoplastic change? *Lancet*, 17 September, 652–4.

Burton, G.R.W. (1992) *Microbiology for the Health Sciences*, 4th edn, J.B. Lippincott Company, London.

Department of Health (1988) *Report of the Working Group to Examine Workloads in Genito Urinary Medicine Clinics* (The Monks Report), Department of Health, London.

Department of Health (1992) *Health of the Nation: Strategy for Health in England*, HMSO, London.

Duncan, I.D. (1992) *Guidelines for Clinical Practice and Management*, NHS Cervical Screening Programme, Hall, Oxford.

Farlow, E. (1993) The cervical smear: a simple test can save a woman's life. *The British Journal of Theatre Nursing*, **2**(11), 4–7.

Held, J.L. (1995) Preventing cervical cancer. *Nursing*, **25**(2), 24.

Moss, T. and Hicks, D. (1994) *The Role of Genito Urinary Medicine Cytology and Colposcopy in Cervical Screening: Does the GU Female Population Merit a Different Cytology/Colposcopy Strategy?* NHS Cervical Screening Programme, Hall, Oxford.

NHS Cervical Screening Programme (1996) *Cervical Screening: A Pocket Guide*, Department of Health, London.

Pike, C. and Chamberlain, J. (1992) *Guidelines on Failsafe Actions*, NHS Cervical Screening Programme, Hall, Oxford.

Robinson, A.J., Mercey, D.E., Preston, M. and Bingham, J.S. (1992) Inflammatory cytology, infection and intraepithelial neoplasia. *International Journal of STD and AIDS*, **3**(2), 123–4.

Royal College of Nursing (1993) *Universal Precautions*, RCN, London.

Royal College of Nursing (1995*)* *Bimanual Pelvic Examination Guidance for Nurses*, RCN, London.

Royal College of Nursing (1996) *Cervical Screening: Guidelines for Good Practice*, RCN, London.

Tang, A., Steadman, T.F., Guinan, E. and Thin, R.N. (1992) Comparative study of two loops used for intraurethral smears in the diagnosis of non-gonococcal urethritis. *Venereology*, **5**, 10–12.

Thorpe, S. (1991) *A Practical Guide to Taking Blood*, Baillière Tindall, London.

United Kingdom Central Council (1992) *Code of Professional Conduct*, UKCC, London.

Young, S.M. and Malet, R.M. (1993) A study comparing cervical cytology results from a genitourinary medicine department with those of two other local populations. *International Journal of STD and AIDS*, **4**(5). 297–9.

FURTHER READING

Dickson, D., Hargie, O. and Morrow, N. (1997) *Communication Skills Training for Health Professionals*, 2nd edn, Stanley Thornes (Publishers) Ltd, Cheltenham.

Index

Page numbers printed in **bold** type refer to figures; those in *italic* to items in the glossary lists